JNĀNA-YOGA

RAMAKRISHNA-VIVEKANANDA CENTER
OF NEW YORK
17 East 94th Street, New York, N.Y. 10028

PUBLICATIONS

By Swami Nikhilananda

HINDUISM: Its Meaning for the Liberation of the Spirit

HOLY MOTHER: Being the Life of Sri Sarada Devi, Wife of Sri Ramakrishna and Helpmate in His Mission

MAN IN SEARCH OF IMMORTALITY: Testimonials from the Hindu Scriptures

VIVEKANANDA: A BIOGRAPHY

Translated by Swami Nikhilananda

THE BHAGAVAD GITA

THE BHAGAVAD GITA (Pocket Edition)

THE GOSPEL OF SRI RAMAKRISHNA

THE GOSPEL OF SRI RAMAKRISHNA (Abridged Edition)

SELF-KNOWLEDGE (Atmabodha)

THE UPANISHADS   Volumes I, II, III, and IV

By Swami Vivekananda

INSPIRED TALKS, My Master and Other Writings

JNANA-YOGA

KARMA-YOGA AND BHAKTI-YOGA

RAJA-YOGA

VIVEKANANDA: THE YOGAS AND OTHER WORKS
(Chosen and with a Biography by Swami Nikhilananda)

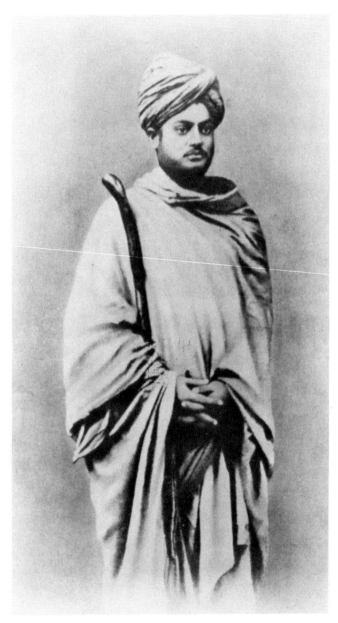

VIVEKANANDA AS A WANDERING MONK

JNĀNA-YOGA

by

SWAMI VIVEKANANDA

REVISED EDITION

new York, December 24, 1994

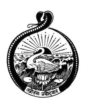

RAMAKRISHNA-VIVEKANANDA CENTER

NEW YORK

JNĀNA-YOGA

Copyright © 1955 by Swami Nikhilananda
Trustee of the Estate of Swami Vivekananda

Printed in the United States of America

FIRST EDITION
(Four Printings)

SECOND EDITION
(Three Printings)

PAPERBACK EDITION 1982

ISBN 0-911206-21-3

Library of Congress Catalog Card Number: 55-8658

PREFACE

The present revised edition of *Jnāna-Yoga* has been taken from *Vivekananda: The Yogas and Other Works,* published in 1953 by the Ramakrishna-Vivekananda Center of New York. The following lines quoted from my preface to the latter will explain the reasons for the editing of the book:

"Swami Vivekananda's public life covered a period of ten years—from 1893, when he appeared at the Parliament of Religions held in Chicago, to 1902, when he gave up his mortal body. These were years of great physical and mental strain as a result of extensive travels, adaptation to new environments, opposition from detractors both in his native land and abroad, incessant public lectures and private instruction, a heavy correspondence, and the organizing of the Ramakrishna Order in India. Hard work and ascetic practices undermined his health. The Swami thus had no time to revise his books, which either were dictated by him or consisted of lectures delivered without notes and taken down in shorthand or longhand. . . . I have therefore felt the need of editing the present collection, making changes wherever they were absolutely necessary, but being always mindful to keep intact the Swami's basic thought."

A few lectures from the earlier edition have been omitted in order to avoid repetition and also to make

v

the present volume uniform with the other **three**
books of the series.

NIKHILANANDA

Ramakrishna-Vivekananda Center
New York
February 21, 1955

CONTENTS

Note on the Pronunciation of Sanskrit and Vernacular Words

a	has	the	sound	of	*o* in *come.*
ā	,,	,,	,,	,,	*a* in *far.*
e	,,	,,	,,	,,	*e* in *bed.*
i	,,	,,	,,	,,	*ee* in *feel.*
o	,,	,,	,,	,,	*o* in *note.*
u	,,	,,	,,	,,	*u* in *full.*
ai, ay	,,	,,	,,	,,	*oy* in *boy.*
au	,,	,,	,,	,,	*o* pronounced deep in the throat.
ch	,,	,,	,,	,,	*ch* in *church.*
ḍ	,,	,,	,,	,,	hard *d* (in English).
g	,,	,,	,,	,,	*g* in *god.*
jn	,,	,,	,,	,,	hard *gy* (in English).
ś	,,	,,	,,	,,	*sh* in *shut.*
th	,,	,,	,,	,,	*t-h* in *boat-house.*

sh may be pronounced as in English.
t and d are soft as in French.

Other consonants appearing in the transliterations may be pronounced as in English.

Diacritical marks have generally not been used in proper names belonging to recent times or in modern and well-known geographical names.

UNIFORM WITH THIS EDITION

Rāja-Yoga
Karma-Yoga and Bhakti-Yoga

JNĀNA-YOGA

THE REAL NATURE OF MAN

(Delivered in London)

G REAT IS THE TENACITY with which man clings to the senses. Yet however substantial he may think the external world in which he lives and moves, there comes a time in the lives of individuals and of races when involuntarily they ask, "Is this real?" To the person who never finds a moment to question the credentials of his senses, whose every moment is occupied with some sort of sense enjoyment—even to him death comes, and he also is compelled to ask, "Is this real?" Religion begins with this question and ends with its answer. Even in the remote past, where recorded history cannot help us—in the mysterious light of mythology, back in the dim twilight of civilization —we find that the same question was asked: "What becomes of this? What is real?"

One of the most poetical of the Upanishads, the *Katha Upanishad,* begins with the inquiry: "When a man dies, there is a dispute: one party declares that he has gone for ever; the other insists that he is still living. Which is the truth?" Various answers have been given. The whole sphere of metaphysics, philosophy, and religion is really filled with various answers to this question. At the same time, attempts have been made to suppress it, to put a stop to the unrest of the mind, which asks: "What is beyond? What is real?" But so long as death remains, all these attempts at suppression will prove unsuccessful. We may talk about seeing nothing beyond and keeping all our hopes and aspirations confined to the present moment, and struggle hard not to think of anything beyond the world of the senses. And perhaps everything outside may help to keep us limited within its narrow bounds; the whole world may combine to prevent us from broadening out beyond the present. Yet, so long as there is death, the question must come again and again: "Is death the end of all these things to which we are clinging, as if they were the most real of all realities, the most substantial of all substances?" The world vanishes in a moment and is gone. Standing on the brink of a precipice beyond which is the infinite, yawning chasm, every mind, however hardened, is bound to recoil and ask, "Is this real?" The hopes of a lifetime, built up little by little with all the energies of a great mind, vanish in a second. Are they real? This question must be answered. Time never lessens its power; on the contrary it adds strength to it.

Then again, there is the desire to be happy. We run after everything to make ourselves happy; we pursue our mad career in the external world of the senses. If you ask the young man with whom life is successful, he will declare that it is real; and he really thinks so. Perhaps, when the same man grows old and finds fortune ever eluding him, he will then declare that this is the result of fate. He finds at last that his desires cannot be fulfilled. Wherever he goes there is an adamantine wall beyond which he cannot pass. Every sense activity results in a reaction. Everything is evanescent. Enjoyment, misery, luxury, wealth, power, and poverty—even life itself—are all evanescent.

Two positions remain to mankind. One is to believe, with the nihilists, that all is nothing, that we know nothing, that we can never know anything about either the future, the past, or even the present. For we must remember that he who denies the past and the future, and wants to stick to the present, is simply a madman. One may as well deny the father and mother and assert the child. It would be equally logical. To deny the past and future, the present must inevitably be denied also. This is one position, that of the nihilists. I have never seen a man who could really become a nihilist for one minute. It is very easy to talk.

Then there is the other position—to seek for an explanation, to seek for the real, to discover in the midst of this eternally changing and evanescent world whatever is real. In this body, which is an aggregate of molecules of matter, is there anything which is real? This has been the search throughout the history of the human mind. In the very oldest times we often find glimpses of light coming into men's minds. We find men even then going a step beyond this body, finding something which is not this external body, although very much like it, something much more complete, much more perfect, which remains even when this body is dissolved. We read in a hymn of the Rig-Veda addressed to the god of fire, who is burning a dead body: "Carry him, Fire, in your arms gently; give him a perfect body, a bright body. Carry him where the fathers live, where there is no more sorrow, where there is no more death."

The same idea we shall find present in every religion, and with it we get another idea. It is a significant
fact that all religions, without one exception, hold that
man is a degeneration of what he was, whether they
clothe this in mythological words, or in the clear
language of philosophy, or in the beautiful expressions
of poetry. This is the one fact that comes out of every
scripture and every mythology: that man as he is, is
a degeneration of what he was. This is the kernel of
truth in the story of Adam's fall in the Jewish scripture. This is again and again repeated in the scriptures
of the Hindus: the dream of a period which they call
the age of truth, when no man died unless he wished
to die, when he could keep his body as long as he
liked, and his mind was pure and strong. There was
no evil, and no misery; and the present age is a corruption of that state of perfection.

Side by side with this, we find everywhere the story
of the deluge. That story itself is a proof that this present age is held by every religion to be a corruption of a
former age. It went on becoming more and more cor-
rupt until the deluge swept away a large portion of
mankind and again the ascending series began. It is
going up slowly again, to reach once more that early
state of purity. You are all aware of the story of the
deluge in the Old Testament. The same story was
current among the ancient Babylonians, the Egyptians,
the Chinese, and the Hindus.

Manu, a great ancient sage, was praying on the
bank of the Ganges, when a little minnow came to
him for protection, and he put it into a pot of water
he had before him. "What do you want?" asked Manu.

The little minnow declared that it was pursued by a bigger fish and wanted protection. Manu carried the little fish home with him. By morning the fish had become as big as the pot and it said, "I cannot live in this pot any longer." Manu put it in a tank, and the next day it was as big as the tank and declared it could not live there any more. So Manu had to take it to a river, and in the morning the fish filled the river. Then Manu put it in the ocean, and it declared: "Manu, I am the Creator of the universe. I have taken this form to come and warn you that I will deluge the world. Build an ark and in it put a pair of every kind of animals, and let your family enter the ark. Out of the water there will project My horn. Fasten the ark to it, and when the deluge subsides, come out and people the earth." So the world was deluged, and Manu saved his own family, and two of every kind of animal, and seeds of every plant. When the deluge subsided he came and peopled the world, and we are all called "man" because we are the progeny of Manu.

Now, human language is the attempt to express the truth that is within. I am fully persuaded that a baby, whose language consists of unintelligible sounds, is attempting to express the highest philosophy; only the baby has not the organs to express it, nor the means. The difference between the language of the highest philosophers and the utterances of babies is one of clarity and not of kind. What you call the most correct, systematic, mathematical language of the present time and the hazy, mystical, mythological language of the ancients differ only in clarity. Both of them have a grand idea behind, which is, as it were, struggling to express itself; and often behind these ancient mythologies are nuggets of truth, while often, I am sorry to say, behind the fine, polished phrases of the moderns is arrant trash. So we need not throw a thing overboard because it is clothed in mythology, because it does not fit in with the notions of Mr. So-and-So or Mrs. So-and-So in modern times. If people should laugh at religion because most religions declared that men must believe in mythologies taught by such and such a prophet, they ought to laugh more at these moderns. In modern times, if a man quotes a Moses or a Buddha or a Christ, he is laughed at; but let him give the name of a Huxley or a Tyndall or a Darwin, and it is swallowed without salt. "Huxley has said it"—that is enough for many. We are free from superstitions indeed! That was a religious superstition, and this a scientific superstition; only in and through that superstition came life-giving ideas of spirituality, whereas in and through this modern superstition come lust and greed. That superstition was worship of God, and this superstition is worship of filthy lucre, of fame, or of power. That is the difference.

To return to mythology. Behind all these stories we find one idea standing supreme: that man is a degeneration of what he was. Coming to the present times, however, we find that modern research seems to repudiate this position absolutely. Evolutionists seem to entirely contradict this assertion. According to them man is the evolution of the mollusc, and therefore what mythology states cannot be true. There in India, however, a mythology which is able to reconcile both these positions. Indian mythology has a theory of cycles: that all movement is in the form of waves. Every rise is attended by a fall, and that by a rise the next moment, that by a fall the next, and that again by another rise. The motion is in cycles. Certainly it is true, even on the grounds of modern research, that man cannot be simply an evolution. Every evolution presupposes an involution. The modern scientific man will tell you that you can only get the amount of energy out of a machine which you have previously put into it. Something cannot be produced out of nothing. If a man is an evolution of the mollusc, then the perfect man, the Buddha-man, the Christ-man must have been involved in the mollusc. If it is not so, whence come these gigantic personalities? Something cannot come out of nothing.

Thus we are in a position to reconcile the scriptures with modern light. That energy which manifests itself slowly through various stages until it becomes the perfect man cannot come out of nothing. It existed somewhere. And if the mollusc or the protoplasm is the first point to which you can trace it, then that protoplasm, somehow or other, must have contained the energy.

There is a great discussion going on as to whether the aggregate of materials we call the body is the cause of the manifestation of the force we call the soul, thought, and so on, or whether it is thought that manifests this body. The religions of the world of course hold that the force called thought manifests the body, and not the reverse. There are schools of modern thought which hold that what we call thought is simply the outcome of the adjustment of the parts of the machine which we call the body. Taking the second position—that the soul or the mass of thought, or whatever you may call it, is the outcome of this machine, the outcome of the chemical and physical combinations of matter making up the body and brain —leaves the question unanswered. What makes the body? What force combines the molecules into the body form? What force is there which takes up material from the mass of matter around it and forms my body one way, another body another way, and so on? What makes these infinite distinctions? To say that the force called the soul is the outcome of the combinations of the molecules of the body is putting the cart before the horse. How did the combinations come? Where was the force to make them? If you say that some other force was the cause of these combinations, and the soul, which is now seen to be combined with a particular mass of matter, is itself the result of the combinations of these material particles —it is no answer. That theory ought to be taken which explains most, if not all, of the facts, without contradicting other existing theories. It is more logical to say that the force which takes up the matter and forms the body is the same which is manifested through that body.

To say, therefore, that the thought-forces manifested in the body are the outcome of the arrangement of molecules and have no independent existence has no meaning. Nor can force evolve out of matter. Rather it is possible to demonstrate that what we call matter does not exist at all. It is only a certain state of force. Solidity, hardness, or any other state of matter can be

proved to be the result of motion. Increase of vortex
motion imparted to fluids gives them the force of solids.
A mass of air in vortex motion, as in a tornado, becomes solid-like and by its impact breaks or cuts
through solids. A thread of a spider's web, if it could
be moved at almost infinite velocity, would be as strong
as an iron chain and would cut through an oak tree.
Looking at it in this way, it would be easier to prove
that what we call matter does not exist. But the other
view cannot be proved.

What is the force which manifests itself through
the body? It is obvious to all of us, whatever that
force be, that it is something which takes particles up,
as it were, and creates forms out of them—human
bodies. None else comes here to manipulate bodies
for you and me. I never saw anybody eat food for me.
I have to assimilate it, manufacture blood and bones
and everything out of that food. What is this mysterious force? Ideas about the future and about the past
seem to be terrifying to many. To many they seem to
be mere speculation. We will take the present as our
theme. What is this force which is now working
through us?

We know how in olden times, in all the ancient
scriptures, this power, this manifestation of power,
was thought to be a bright substance having the form
of this body, which remained even after the body fell.
Later on, however, we find a higher idea coming: that
this bright body did not represent the force. Whatsoever has form, it was discovered, must be the result
of combinations of particles and requires something
else behind it to move it. If this body requires some-

thing which is not the body to manipulate it, the
bright body, by the same necessity, will also require
something other than itself to manipulate it. That
something was called the Soul—the Ātman, in Sanskrit. It was the Ātman which through the bright body,
as it were, worked on the gross body outside. The
bright body is considered as the receptacle of the mind,
and the Ātman is beyond that. It is not even the mind;
it works the mind, and through the mind, the body.
You have an Ātman, I have another; each one of us
has a separate Ātman and a separate fine body, and
through that we work on the gross external body.
Questions were then asked about this Ātman, about
its nature. What is this Ātman, this Soul of man,
which is neither the body nor the mind? Great discussions followed. Speculations were made, various
shades of philosophic inquiry came into existence. I
shall try to place before you some of the conclusions
that have been reached about this Ātman.

The different philosophies seem to agree that this
Ātman, whatever it may be, has neither form nor
shape; and that which has neither form nor shape
must be omnipresent. Time begins with mind; space
also is in the mind. Causation cannot stand without
time—without the idea of succession there cannot be
any idea of causation. Time, space, and causation,
therefore, are in the mind; and as this Ātman is beyond the mind and formless, it must be beyond time,
beyond space, and beyond causation. Now, if it is
beyond time, space, and causation, it must be infinite.
Then comes the highest speculation in our philosophy.
The infinite cannot be two. If the Soul be infinite,

there can be only one Soul, and all ideas of various souls—of your having one soul, and I having another, and so forth—are not real. The Real Man therefore is one and infinite, the omnipresent Spirit. And the apparent man is only a limitation of that Real Man. In that sense the mythologies are true in saying that the apparent man, however great he may be, is only a dim reflection of the Real Man, who is beyond. The Real Man, the Spirit, being beyond cause and effect, not bound by time and space, must therefore be free. He was never bound and could not be bound. The apparent man, the reflection, is limited by time, space, and causation, and is therefore bound. Or in the language of some of our philosophers, he appears to be bound but really is not. This is the reality behind our souls, this omnipresence, this spiritual nature, this infinity. The soul is infinite. Therefore there is no question of birth and death.

Some children were being examined. The examiner put to them rather hard questions, and among them was this one: "Why does not the earth fall?" He wanted to evoke answers about gravitation. Most of the children could not answer at all; a few answered that it was gravitation or something. One bright little girl answered it by putting another question: "Where should it fall?" The first question is nonsense. Where should the earth fall? There is no falling or rising for the earth. In infinite space there is no up or down; up and down are only in the relative. Where is any going or coming for the infinite? Whence should it come and whither should it go?

Thus, when people cease to think of the past or

future, when they give up the idea of body because
the body comes and goes and is limited, then they
have risen to a higher ideal. The body is not the Real
Man; neither is the mind, for the mind waxes and
wanes. It is the Spirit beyond, which alone can live
for ever. The body and mind are continually changing
and are, in fact, only names of series of changeful
phenomena, like rivers whose waters are in a constant
state of flux, yet present the appearance of unbroken
streams. Every particle in this body is continually
changing; no one has the same body for many minutes
together, and yet we think of it as the same body. So
with the mind: one moment it is happy, another
moment unhappy; one moment strong, another weak
—an ever changing whirlpool. That cannot be the
Spirit, which is infinite. Change can only be in the
limited. To say that the infinite changes in any way
is absurd; it cannot be. You can move and I can move,
as limited bodies; every particle in this universe is in
a state of flux; but taking the universe as a unit, as
one whole, it cannot move, it cannot change. Motion
is always a relative thing. I move in relation to something else. Any particle in this universe can change
in relation to any other particle. But take the whole
universe as one; then in relation to what can it move?
There is nothing besides it. So this infinite Unit is
unchangeable, immovable, absolute, and this is the
Real Man. Our reality, therefore, consists in the Universal, and not in the limited. This is an old delusion,
however comfortable it may be—to think that we are
little limited beings, constantly changing.

People are frightened when they are told they are

Universal Being, everywhere present. "Through everything you work, through every foot you move, through
every lip you talk, through every heart you feel."
People are frightened when they are told this. They
will again and again ask you if they are not going to
keep their individuality. What is individuality? I
should like to see it. A baby has no moustache; when
he grows to be a man, perhaps he has a moustache
and beard. His individuality would be lost if it were
in the body. If I lose one eye or if I lose one of my
hands, my individuality would be lost if it were in the
body. Then a drunkard should not give up drinking,
because he would lose his individuality. A thief should
not be a good man, because he would thereby lose his
individuality. Indeed, no man ought to change his
habits, for fear of this. Nor can individuality be in
memory. Suppose, on account of a blow on the head,
I forget all about my past; then I have lost all individuality, I am gone. I do not remember two or three
years of my childhood, and if memory and existence
are one, then whatever I forget is gone. That part of
my life which I do not remember, I did not live. That
is a very narrow idea of individuality.

There is no individuality except in the Infinite.
That is the only condition which does not change.
Everything else is in a state of flux. We are not individuals yet. We are struggling towards individuality;
and that is the Infinite. That is the real nature of
man. He alone lives whose life is in the whole universe;
the more we concentrate our lives on limited things,
the faster we go towards death. Those moments alone
we live when our lives are in the universe, in others;

and living this little life is death, simply death, and
that is why the fear of death comes. The fear of death
can only be conquered when a man realizes that so long
as there is one life in this universe, he is living. When
he can say, "I am in everything, in everybody; I am
in all lives; I am the universe," then alone comes the
state of fearlessness. To talk of immortality in constantly changing things is absurd. Says an old Sanskrit
philosopher: "It is only the Spirit that is the individual,
because It is infinite." Infinity cannot be divided; infinity cannot be broken into pieces. It is the same one
undivided unit for ever; and this is the individual
man, the Real Man. The apparent man is merely a
struggle to express, to manifest, this individuality which
is beyond. Evolution is not in the Spirit.

These changes which are going on—the wicked
becoming good, the animal becoming man; take them
in whatever way you like—are not in the Spirit. They
are the evolution of nature and the manifestation of
the Spirit. Suppose there is a screen hiding you from
me, in which there is a small hole through which I
can see some of the faces before me, just a few faces.
Now suppose the hole begins to grow larger and larger,
and as it does so, more and more of the scene before
me reveals itself; when at last the whole screen has
disappeared, I stand face to face with you all. You did
not change at all; it was the hole that was evolving,
and you were gradually manifesting yourselves. So it
is with the Spirit. No perfection is going to be attained.
You are already free and perfect.

What are these ideas of religion and God and
searching for the hereafter? Why does man look for a
God? Why does man, in every nation, in every state

of society, want a perfect ideal somewhere, either in
man, in God, or elsewhere? Because that idea is within
you. It was your own heart beating and you did not
know; you were mistaking it for something external.
It is the God within your own self that is impelling
you to seek Him, to realize Him. After long searches
here and there, in temples and in churches, on earth
and in heaven, at last you come back to your own
soul, completing the circle from where you started,
and find that He whom you have been seeking all
over the world, for whom you have been weeping and
praying in churches and temples, on whom you were
looking as the mystery of all mysteries, shrouded in
the clouds, is the nearest of the near, is your own
Self, the reality of your life, body, and soul.[1]

[1] Non-dualistic Vedānta speaks of two souls, as it were:
the Real Soul and the apparent soul, the Universal and the
individual, the Absolute and the phenomenal. The Real
Soul, which is the same as Brahman, is Pure Consciousness, birthless, deathless, and beyond time, space, and the
law of causation. The apparent soul is the one with which
we deal in our daily practical life, which identifies itself
with the body, senses, and mind, and is subject to birth,
death, and other phenomenal changes. In reality there is
only one Existence, designated as Brahman. Through
māyā, or metaphysical ignorance, the apparent multiplicity
is created and Brahman appears as the individual soul and
the universe. By means of spiritual discipline the individual
soul ultimately recognizes its oneness with the Universal
Soul. Throughout this book the word *soul*, when it denotes Brahman, or Pure Consciousness, has been spelt
with a capital *s*; when it denotes the individual soul it has
been spelt with a small *s*, except in a few instances, where,
in order to emphasize the soul's potential divine nature,
it has been spelt with a capital. The same applies to the
word *self*.

That Self is your own nature. Assert It, manifest It. You are not to become pure; you are pure already. You are not to become perfect; you are that already. Nature is like a screen which is hiding the reality beyond. Every good thought that you think or act upon simply tears the veil, as it were, and the Purity, the Infinity, the God behind, is manifested more and more. This is the whole history of man. Finer and finer becomes the veil, more and more of the light behind shines forth; for it is its nature to shine.

That Self cannot be known; in vain we try to know It. Were It knowable, It would not be what It is; for It is the eternal Subject. Knowledge is a limitation; knowledge is an objectification. It is the eternal Subject of everything, the eternal Witness of this universe —your own Self. Knowledge is, as it were, a lower step, a degeneration. We are that eternal Subject already; how can we know It?

The infinite Self is the real nature of every man, and he is struggling to express It in various ways. Otherwise, why are there so many ethical codes? Where is the explanation of all ethics? One idea stands out as the centre of all ethical systems, expressed in various forms—namely, doing good to others. The guiding motive of mankind should be charity towards men, charity towards all animals. But these are all various expressions of that eternal truth that "I am the universe; this universe is one." Or else, where is the explanation? Why should I do good to my fellow men? Why should I do good to others? What compels me? It is sympathy, the feeling of sameness everywhere. The hardest hearts sometimes feel sympathy for other beings. Even the man who gets frightened if he is told that this assumed individuality is really a delusion, that it is ignoble to try to cling to this apparent individuality—that very man will tell you that extreme self-abnegation is the centre of all morality. And what is perfect self-abnegation? It means the abnegation of this apparent self, the abnegation of all selfishness.

This idea of "me" and "mine"—ahamkāra and mamatā—is the result of past superstition, and the more this present self passes away, the more the Real Self becomes manifest. This is true self-abnegation, the centre, the basis, the gist of all moral teaching, and whether man knows it or not, the whole world is slowly going towards it, practising it more or less. Only, the vast majority of mankind are doing it unconsciously. Let them do it consciously. Let them make the sacrifice, knowing that "me" and "mine" are not the Real Self, but only a limitation. But one glimpse of that infinite Reality which is behind, but one spark of that infinite Fire which is the All, represents the present man. The Infinite is his true nature.

What is the utility, the effect, the result of this knowledge? In these days we have to measure everything by utility—by how many pounds, shillings, and pence it represents. What right has a person to ask that truth should be judged by the standard of utility or money? Suppose there is no utility, will it be less true? Utility is not the test of truth. Nevertheless, there is the highest utility in this. Happiness, we see, is what everyone is seeking for; but the majority seek it in things which are evanescent and not real. No

happiness was ever found in the senses. There never
was a person who found happiness in the senses or in
enjoyment of the senses. Happiness is found only in
the Spirit. Therefore the highest utility for mankind
is to find this happiness in the Spirit.

The next point is that ignorance is the great mother
of all misery, and the fundamental ignorance is to
think that the Infinite weeps and cries, that It is
finite. This is the basis of all ignorance—that we, the
immortal, the ever pure, the perfect Spirit, think we
are little minds, we are little bodies. It is the mother
of all selfishness. As soon as I think I am a little body,
I want to preserve it, to protect it, to keep it nice, at
the expense of other bodies. Then you and I become
separate. As soon as this idea of separation comes, it
opens the door to all mischief and leads to all misery.
This, then, is the utility of this knowledge—that if a
small fractional part of the human beings living today
can put aside the idea of selfishness, narrowness, and
littleness, this earth will become a paradise tomorrow.
But with machines and improvements of material
knowledge only, it will never be so. These only increase misery, as oil poured on fire increases the flame
all the more. Without the knowledge of the Spirit, all
material knowledge is only adding fuel to fire, only
giving into the hands of selfish man one more instrument to take what belongs to others, to live upon the
life of others instead of giving up his life for them.

Is it practical?—is another question. Can it be practised in modern society? Truth does not pay homage to
any society, ancient or modern. Society has to pay
homage to truth or die. Societies should be moulded

upon truth; truth has not to adjust itself to society. If such a noble truth as unselfishness cannot be practised in society, it is better for a man to give up society and go into the forest. That is the daring man.

There are two sorts of courage. One is the courage of facing the cannon; and the other is the courage of spiritual conviction. An emperor who invaded India was told by his teacher to go and see some of the sages there. After a long search for one, he found a very old man sitting on a block of stone. The emperor talked with him a little and became very much impressed by his wisdom. He asked the sage to go to his country with him. "No," said the sage, "I am quite satisfied with my forest here." Said the emperor: "I will give you money, position, wealth. I am the emperor of the world." "No," replied the man, "I don't care for those things." The emperor replied, "If you do not go, I will kill you." The man smiled serenely and said: "That is the most foolish thing you ever said, Emperor. You cannot kill me. Me the wind cannot dry, fire cannot burn, sword cannot kill; for I am the birthless, the deathless, the ever living, omnipotent, omnipresent Spirit." This is spiritual boldness, while the other is the courage of a lion or a tiger.

During the Mutiny of 1857, there was a Swami, a very great soul, whom a Mohammedan mutineer stabbed severely. The Hindu mutineers caught and brought the man to the Swami, offering to kill him. But the Swami looked up calmly and said, "My brother, thou art He, thou art He!" and expired. This is another instance.

What good is it to talk of the strength of your muscles, of the superiority of your Western institutions, if you cannot make truth square with your society, if you cannot build up a society into which the highest truth will fit? What is the good of this boastful talk about your grandeur and greatness if you stand up and say, "This courage is not practical"? Is nothing practical but pounds, shillings, and pence? If so, why boast of your society? That society is the greatest where the highest truths become practical. That is my opinion. And if society is not fit for the highest truths, make it so—and the sooner, the better.

Stand up, men and women, in this spirit, dare to believe in the truth, dare to practise the truth! The world requires a few hundred bold men and women. Practise that boldness which dares know the truth, which dares show the truth in life, which does not quake before death, nay, welcomes death, makes a man know that he is the Spirit, that in the whole universe nothing can kill him. Then you will be free. Then you will know your real Soul.

"This Ātman is first to be heard of, then thought about, and then meditated upon." There is a great tendency in modern times to talk too much of work and decry thought. Doing is very good, but that comes from thinking. Little manifestations of energy through the muscles are called work. But where there is no thought, there will be no work. Fill the brain, therefore, with high thoughts, with the highest ideals; place them day and night before you, and out of that will come great work. Talk not about impurity, but say that we are pure. We have hypnotized ourselves into this thought that we are little, that we are born and

that we are going to die, and into a constant state
of fear.

There is a story about a lioness who was big with
young. Going about in search of prey, and seeing a
flock of sheep, she jumped upon them. She died in
the effort and a little baby lion was born, motherless.
It was taken care of by the sheep and they brought it
up. It grew up with them, ate grass, and bleated like
the sheep. And although in time it became a big full-
grown lion, it thought it was a sheep. One day another
lion came in search of prey and was astonished to find
that in the midst of this flock of sheep was a lion,
fleeing like the sheep at the approach of danger. He
tried to get near the sheep-lion to tell it that it was not
a sheep but a lion, but the poor animal fled at his
approach. However, he watched his opportunity and
one day found the sheep-lion sleeping. He approached
it and said, "You are a lion." "I am a sheep," cried
the other lion; it could not believe the contrary, but
bleated. The lion dragged it towards a lake and said,
"Look here: there is my reflection and there is yours."
Then came the comparison. The sheep-lion looked at
the lion and then at its own reflection, and in a moment came the idea that it was a lion. The lion roared;
the bleating was gone.

You are lions; you are the Soul, pure, infinite, and
perfect. The might of the universe is within you.
"Why weepest thou, my friend? There is neither birth
nor death for thee. Why weepest thou? There is no
disease or misery for thee. Thou art like the infinite
sky: clouds of various colours come over it, play for a

moment, then vanish; but the sky is ever the same eternal blue."

Why do we see wickedness? There was a stump of a tree, and in the dark a thief came that way and said, "That is a policeman." A young man waiting for his beloved saw it and thought it was his sweetheart. A child who had been told ghost stories took it for a ghost and began to shriek. But all the time it was the stump of a tree. We see the world as we are. Suppose there is a baby in a room with a bag of gold on the table, and a thief comes and steals the gold. Would the baby know it was stolen? That which we have inside, we see outside. The baby has no thief inside and sees no thief outside. So with all knowledge.

Do not talk of the wickedness of the world and all its sins. Weep that you are bound to see wickedness yet. Weep that you are bound to see sin everywhere. If you want to help the world, do not condemn it. Do not weaken it more. For what is sin and what is misery —what are all these but the results of weakness? The world is made weaker and weaker every day by such teachings. Men are taught from childhood that they are weak and sinners. Teach them that they are all glorious children of immortality, even those who are the weakest in manifestation. Let positive, strong, helpful thoughts enter into their brains from very childhood. Lay yourselves open to these thoughts, and not to weakening and paralysing ones. Say to your own minds, "I am He, I am He." Let it ring day and night in your minds like a song, and at the point of death declare, "I am He." That is the truth. The infinite strength of the world is yours. Drive out the superstition that has covered your minds. Let us be brave. Know the truth and practise the truth. The goal may be distant, but awake, arise, and stop not till the goal is reached.

MĀYĀ

(*Delivered in London*)

A<small>LMOST ALL OF</small> Y<small>OU</small> have heard of the word *māyā*. Generally it is used, though incorrectly, to denote illusion or delusion or some such thing. But the theory of māyā forms one of the pillars upon which Vedānta rests; it is therefore necessary that it should be properly understood. I ask a little patience of you, for there is a great danger of its being misunderstood.

The oldest use of *māyā* that we find in Vedic literature is in the sense of delusion; but then the real theory had not been reached. We find such passages as, "Indra through his māyā assumed various forms." Here, it is true, the word *māyā* means something like magic, and we find various other passages where it always takes the same meaning. The word *māyā* then dropped out of sight altogether. But in the meantime the idea was developing. Later the question was raised: "Why can't we know the secret of the universe?" And the answer given was very significant: "Because we talk in vain, and because we are satisfied with the things of the senses, and because we are running after desires, therefore we cover the Reality, as it were, with a mist." Here the word *māyā* is not used at all; but we get the idea that the cause of our ignorance is a kind of mist that has come between us and the truth. Much later on, in one of the latest Upanishads, we find the word *māyā* reappearing; but by this time a transformation had taken place in it and a mass of new meaning had attached itself to the word. Theories had been propounded and repeated, others had been taken up, until at last the idea of māyā became fixed. We read in the *Śvetāśvatara Upanishad*: "Know nature to be māyā, and the Ruler of this māyā, the Lord Himself."

Coming to later philosophers, we find that this word *māyā* was manipulated in various fashions, until we come to the great Śankarāchārya. The theory of māyā was manipulated a little by the Buddhists, too, but in the hands of the Buddhists it became very much like what is called idealism, and that is the meaning which is now generally given to the word *māyā*.

When the Hindu says the world is māyā, at once people get the idea that the world is an illusion. This interpretation has some basis, as coming through the Buddhist philosophers, because there was one section of those philosophers who did not believe in the external world at all. But the māyā of Vedānta, in its final form, is neither idealism nor realism, nor is it a theory. It is a simple statement of fact—what we are and what we see around us.

As I have told you before, the minds of the people from whom the Vedas came were intent upon following principles, discovering principles. They had no time to work upon details or to wait for them; they wanted to go deep into the heart of things. Something beyond was calling them, as it were, and they could not wait. In the Upanishads we find that the details of subjects which are now dealt with by science are often very erroneous, but at the same time the princi-

ples are correct. For instance, the idea of ether, which
is one of the latest theories of modern science, is to be
found in our ancient literature in a form much more
developed than is the modern scientific theory of ether
today. But it was only a principle. When the Vedic
thinkers tried to demonstrate that principle, they made
many mistakes. The theory of the all-pervading life
principle, of which all lives in this universe are but
differing manifestations, was understood in Vedic
times; it is found in the Brāhmanas. There is a long
hymn in one of the Samhitās in praise of Prāna, of
which all life is but a manifestation. By the bye, it
may interest some of you to know that there are theories in the Vedic philosophy about the origin of life
on this earth, very similar to those which have been
advanced by some modern European scientists. You
of course all know that there is a theory that life came
from other planets. It was a settled doctrine with some
Vedic philosophers that life came, in this way, from
the moon.

We find these Vedic thinkers very courageous and
wonderfully bold in propounding large and generalized
theories. Their solution of the mystery of the universe,
from the analysis of the external world, was as satisfactory as it could be. The detailed workings of modern science do not bring the question one step nearer
to solution, because the principles propounded by the
Vedic thinkers failed. If the theory of ether failed in
ancient times to give a solution of the mystery of the
universe, working out the details of that ether theory
will not bring us much nearer to the truth. If the
theory of all-pervading life failed as a theory of this

universe, it will not mean anything more if worked out in detail; for the details do not change the principles of the universe. What I mean is that, in their inquiry into the principles, the Hindu thinkers were as bold as, and in some cases much bolder than, the moderns. They made some of the grandest generalizations that have yet been reached, and some of these still remain as theories which modern science has yet to arrive at, even as theories. For instance, they not only arrived at the ether theory, but went beyond and classified mind, also, as a still more rarefied ether. Beyond that, again, they found a still more rarefied ether. Yet that was no solution; it did not solve the problem. No amount of knowledge of the external world could solve the problem.

"But," says the scientist, "we are just beginning to know a little; wait a few thousand years and we shall get the solution." "No," says the Vedāntist; for he has proved beyond all doubt that the mind is limited, that it cannot go beyond certain limits—beyond time, space, and causation. As no man can jump out of his own self, so no man can go beyond the limits that have been put upon him by the laws of time and space. Every attempt to solve the laws of causation, time, and space is futile, because the very attempt can only be made by taking for granted the existence of these three.

What, then, does the statement that the world exists mean? It really means that the world has no existence. What, again, does the statement that the world has no existence mean? It means that it has no absolute existence: it exists only in relation to my mind, to your

mind, and to the mind of everyone else. We see this
world with the five senses, but if we had another sense,
we would see in it something more. If we had yet
another sense, it would appear as something still different. It has, therefore, no real existence; it has no unchangeable, immovable, infinite existence. Nor can it
be said to have non-existence, since it exists and we
have to work in and through it. It is a mixture of
existence and non-existence.

Coming from abstractions to the common, everyday
details of our lives, we find that our whole life is a
mixture of this contradiction of existence and non-
existence. There is this contradiction in knowledge:
It seems that man can know everything if he only
wants to know; but before he has gone a few steps he
finds an adamantine wall which he cannot pass. All
his work is in a circle, and he cannot go beyond that
circle. The problems which are nearest and dearest to
him are impelling him on and calling, day and night,
for a solution; but he cannot solve them, because he
cannot go beyond this intellect. We know that desire
is implanted strongly in man. Again, we know that the
only good is to be obtained by controlling and checking it. With our every breath, every impulse of our
heart asks us to be selfish; at the same time, there is
some power beyond us which says that it is unselfishness alone which is good. Every child is a born optimist; he dreams golden dreams. In youth he becomes
still more optimistic. It is hard for a young man to
believe that there is such a thing as death, such a thing
as defeat or degradation. Old age comes, and life is a
mass of ruins. Dreams have vanished into the air, and

the man becomes a pessimist. Thus we go from one extreme to another, buffeted by nature, without knowing where we are going.

I am reminded of a celebrated song in the *Lalita Vistara*, a biography of Buddha. Buddha was born, says the book, as the Saviour of mankind, but he forgot himself in the luxuries of his palace. Some angels came and sang a song to rouse him. And the burden of the whole song is that we are floating down the river of life, which is continually changing, with no stop and no rest. What, then, are we to do? The man who has enough to eat and drink is an optimist, and he avoids all mention of misery, for it frightens him. Tell not him of the sorrows and the sufferings of the world; go to him and tell that it is all good. "Yes, I am safe," says he. "Look at me, I have a nice house to live in; I do not fear cold and hunger. Therefore do not bring these horrible pictures before me." But on the other hand there are others dying of cold and hunger. If you go and teach *them* that it is all good, they will not hear. How can they wish others to be happy when they are miserable? Thus we are oscillating between optimism and pessimism.

Then there is the tremendous fact of death. The whole world is going towards death. Everything dies. All our progress, our vanities, our reforms, our luxuries, our wealth, our knowledge, have that one end— death. That is all that is certain. Cities come and go, empires rise and fall, planets break into pieces and crumble into dust, to be blown about by the atmospheres of other planets. Thus it has been going on from time without beginning. Death is the end of everything. Death is the end of life, of beauty, of wealth, of power, of virtue too. Saints die and sinners die, kings die and beggars die. They are all going to death. And yet this tremendous clinging to life exists. Somehow, we do not know why, we cling to life; we cannot give it up. And this is māyā.

A mother is nursing her child with great care; all her soul, her life, is in that child. The child grows, becomes a man, and perchance becomes a blackguard and a brute, kicks her and beats her every day; and yet the mother clings to the child, and when her reason awakes, she covers it all up with the idea of love. She little thinks that it is not love, but something else, which has got hold of her nerves and which she cannot shake off. However she may try, she cannot shake off the bondage she is in. And this is māyā.

We are all running after the golden fleece. Every one of us thinks that it will be his. Every reasonable man sees that his chance is perhaps one in twenty millions, yet everyone struggles for it. And this is māyā.

Death is stalking day and night over this earth of ours, but at the same time we think we shall live eternally. A question was once asked of King Yudhishthira: "What is the most wonderful thing on this earth?" And the king replied, "Every day people are dying around us, and yet men think they will never die." And this is māyā.

These tremendous contradictions in our intellect, in our knowledge, indeed, in all the facts of our life, face us on all sides. A reformer arises and wants to remedy the evils existing in a certain nation; and before they have been remedied, a thousand other evils arise in another place. It is like an old house that is falling: you patch it up in one place and the ruin extends to another. In India our reformers cry and preach against the evils of enforced widowhood. In the West, non-marriage is the great evil. Help the unmarried on one side; they are suffering. Help the widows on the other; *they* are suffering. It is like chronic rheumatism: you drive it from the head and it goes to the body; you drive it from there and it goes to the feet. Reformers arise and preach that learning, wealth, and culture should not be in the hands of a select few; and they do their best to make them accessible to all. These may bring more happiness to some, but perhaps, as culture grows, physical happiness lessens. The knowledge of happiness brings the knowledge of unhappiness. Which way, then, shall we go? The least amount of material prosperity that we enjoy is elsewhere causing the same amount of misery. This is the law. The young, perhaps, do not see it clearly, but those who have lived long enough and those who have struggled enough will understand it. And this is māyā.

These things are going on, day and night, and to find a solution of this problem is impossible. Why should it be so? It is impossible to answer this, because the question cannot be logically formulated. There is neither *how* nor *why* in fact; we only know that it *is* and that we cannot help it. Even to grasp it, to draw an exact image of it in our own mind, is beyond our power. How can we solve it, then?

Māyā is a statement of the fact of this universe, of how it is going on. People generally get frightened

when they are told about these things. But bold we
must be. Hiding facts is not the way to find a remedy.
As you all know, a hare hunted by dogs puts its head
down and thinks itself safe. When we take refuge in
optimism we act just like the hare. But that is no
remedy. There are objections to this idea, but you
may remark that they are generally from people who
possess many of the good things of life. In this country
[England] it is very difficult to become a pessimist.
Everyone tells me how wonderfully the world is going
on, how progressive it is. But what he himself is, is
his own world. The same old questions arise again and
again. People assert that Christianity must be the only
true religion of the world, because the Christian nations are prosperous! But that assertion contradicts
itself, because the prosperity of the Christian nations
depends on the misfortune of non-Christian nations.
There must be some to prey on. Suppose the whole
world were to become Christian; then the Christian
nations would become poor, because there would be
no non-Christian nations for them to prey upon. Thus
the argument kills itself. Animals are living upon
plants, men upon animals, and, worst of all, upon one
another—the strong upon the weak. This is going on
everywhere. And this is māyā.

What solution do you find for this? We hear every
day many explanations and are told that in the long
run all will be good. Taking it for granted that this is
possible, why should there be this diabolical way of
doing good? Why cannot good be done through good,
instead of through these diabolical methods? The
descendants of the human beings of today will be

happy; but why must there be all this suffering now? There is no solution. And this is māyā.

Again, we often hear that one of the features of evolution is that it gradually eliminates evil from the world, until evil is completely eliminated, when at last only good will remain. That is very nice to hear; it panders to the vanity of those who have enough of this world's goods, who have no hard struggle to face every day and are not being crushed under the wheel of this so-called evolution. It is very good and comforting indeed to such fortunate ones. The common herd may suffer, but they do not care; let the rest die— they are of no consequence. Very good. Yet this argument is fallacious from beginning to end. It takes for granted, in the first place, that manifested good and evil in this world are two absolute realities. In the second place, it makes a still worse assumption: that the amount of good is an increasing quantity, and the amount of evil is a decreasing quantity. So if evil is being eliminated in this way, by what is called evolution, there will come a time when all this evil will be eliminated and what remains will be all good. Very easy to say, but can it be proved that evil is a lessening quantity?

Take, for instance, the man who lives in a forest, who does not know how to cultivate the mind, cannot read a book, has not heard of such a thing as writing. If he is severely wounded, he is soon all right again, while we die if we get a scratch. Again, machines are making things cheap, making for progress and evolution, but millions are crushed that one may become rich—thousands at the same time become poorer and poorer, and whole masses of human beings are made slaves. That is the way it is going on.

The animal man lives in the senses. If he does not get enough to eat, he is miserable, or if something happens to his body, he is miserable. In the senses both his misery and his happiness begin and end. As soon as this man progresses, as soon as his horizon of happiness increases, his horizon of unhappiness increases proportionately. The man in the forest does not know what it is to be jealous, to be in the law-courts, to pay taxes, to be blamed by society, and to be ruled over day and night by the most tremendous tyranny that human diabolism ever invented, which pries into the secrets of every human heart. He does not know that man becomes a thousand times more diabolical than any other animal, with all his vain knowledge and with all his pride. Thus it is that, as we emerge out of the senses, we develop higher powers of enjoyment, and at the same time we develop higher powers of suffering too. The nerves become finer and capable of more suffering. In every society we often find that the ignorant common man, when abused, does not feel much, but he feels a good thrashing. But the gentleman cannot bear a single word of abuse: he has become so finely nerved; his misery has increased with his susceptibility to happiness. This does not go far to prove the evolutionist's case.

As we increase our power to be happy we also increase our power to suffer, and sometimes I am inclined to think that if we increase our power to become happy in arithmetical progression, we shall increase, on the other hand, our power to become miserable in geometrical progression. We who are progressing know that the more we progress, the more avenues are opened to pain as well as to pleasure. And this is māyā.

Thus we find that māyā is not a theory for the explanation of the world; it is simply a statement of facts as they exist—that the very basis of our being is contradiction, that everywhere we have to move through this tremendous contradiction, that wherever there is good, there must also be evil, and wherever there is evil there must be some good, wherever there is life, death must follow as its shadow, and everyone who smiles will have to weep, and whoever weeps must smile also. Nor can this state of things be remedied. We may vainly imagine that there will be a place where there will be only good, and no evil, where we shall only smile and never weep. This is impossible in the very nature of things; for the conditions will remain the same. Wherever there is the power of producing a smile in us, there lurks the power of producing tears. Wherever there is the power of producing happiness, there lurks somewhere the power of making us miserable.

Thus the Vedānta philosophy is neither optimistic nor pessimistic. It voices both these views and takes things as they are; it admits that this world is a mixture of good and evil, happiness and misery, and that to increase the one must of necessity increase the other. There will never be a perfectly good or bad world, because the very idea is a contradiction in terms. The great secret revealed by this analysis is that good and bad are not two cut-and-dried, separate existences. There is not one thing in this world of ours

which you can label as good, and good alone; and
there is not one thing in the universe which you can
label as bad, and bad alone. The very same phenomenon which is appearing to be good now may appear to
be bad tomorrow. The same thing which is producing
misery in one may produce happiness in another. The
fire that burns the child may cook a good meal for a
starving man. The same nerves that carry the sensations of misery carry also the sensations of happiness.

The only way to stop evil, therefore, is to stop good
also; there is no other way. To stop death we shall
have to stop life also. Life without death and happiness without misery are contradictions, and neither
can be found alone, because both of them are different
manifestations of the same thing.

What I thought to be good yesterday, I do not think
to be good now. When I look back upon my life and
see what were my ideals at different times, I find this
to be so. At one time my ideal was to drive a strong
pair of horses; at another time I thought if I could
make a certain kind of sweetmeat I should be perfectly happy; later I imagined that I should be entirely
satisfied if I had a wife and children and plenty of
money. Today I laugh at all these ideals as mere childish nonsense. Vedānta says that there must come a
time when we shall look back and laugh at the ideas
which make us afraid of giving up our individuality.
Each one of us wants to keep this body for an in-
definite time, thinking he will be very happy; but
there will come a time when we shall laugh at this
idea.

Now, if such be the truth, we are in a state of

hopeless contradiction—neither existence nor non-existence, neither misery nor happiness, but a mixture of them. What, then, is the use of Vedānta and all other philosophies and religions? And above all, what is the use of doing good work? This is a question that comes to the mind. If it is true that you cannot do good without doing evil, and that whenever you try to create happiness there will always be misery, people will ask you, "What is the use of doing good?" The answer is, in the first place, that we must work for lessening misery, for that is the only way to make ourselves happy. Every one of us finds it out sooner or later in life. The bright ones find it out a little earlier, and the dull ones a little later. The dull ones pay very dearly for the discovery, and the bright ones less dearly. In the second place, we must do our part, because that is the only way of getting out of this life of contradiction. The forces of good and evil will keep the universe alive for us until we awake from our dreams and give up this making of mud-pies. That lesson we shall have to learn, and it will take a long, long time to learn it.

Attempts have been made in Germany to build a system of philosophy on the basis that the Infinite has become the finite. Such attempts are also made in England. The analysis of the position of these philosophers is this: that the Infinite is trying to express Itself in this universe, and that there will come a time when the Infinite will succeed in doing so. This is all very well, and we have used the words *Infinite* and *manifestation* and *expression,* and so on; but philosophers naturally ask for a logical, irrefutable basis for the statement that the finite can fully express the Infinite. The Absolute or the Infinite can become this universe only by limitation. Everything must be limited that comes through the senses or through the mind or through the intellect; and for the limited to be unlimited is simply absurd; it can never be.

Vedānta, on the other hand, says that it is true that the Absolute or the Infinite is trying to express Itself in the finite, but there will come a time when It will find that it is impossible, and It will then have to beat a retreat; and this beating a retreat means renunciation, which is the real beginning of religion. Nowadays it is very hard even to talk of renunciation. It was said of me in America that I was a man who came out of a land that talked of renunciation and had been dead and buried for five thousand years. So says perhaps the English philosopher. Yet it is true that that is the only path to religion. Renounce and give up. What did Christ say? "He that loseth his life for my sake shall find it." Again and again did he preach renunciation as the only way to perfection.

There comes a time when the mind awakes from this long and dreary dream, the child gives up its play and wants to go back to its mother. It finds the truth of the statement: "Desire is never satisfied by the enjoyment of desires; it only increases the more, like fire when butter is poured upon it." This is true of all sense enjoyments, all intellectual enjoyments, and all the enjoyments of which the human mind is capable. They are nothing; they are within māyā, within this network which we cannot get out of. We may run about therein through infinite time and yet find no

escape, and whenever we struggle to get a little enjoyment a mass of misery falls upon us. How awful this
is! And when I think of it I cannot but consider that
this theory of māyā, this statement that it is all māyā,
is the best and only explanation.

What an amount of misery there is in this world!
And if you travel among various nations you will find
that one nation attempts to cure its evils by one means,
and another by another. The very same evil has been
taken up by various races, and attempts have been
made in various ways to check it; yet no nation has
succeeded. If it has been minimized at one point, a
mass of evil has been crowded in at another point.
Thus it goes.

The Hindus, to keep up a high standard of chastity
in the race, have sanctioned child-marriage, which in
the long run has degraded the race. At the same time,
I cannot deny that this child-marriage makes the race
more chaste. What would you have? If you want the
nation to be more chaste, you weaken men and women
physically by child-marriage. On the other hand, are
you in England any better off? No, because chastity
is the life of a nation. Do you not find in history that
the first death-sign of a nation has been unchastity?
When that has entered, the end of the race is in sight.
Where shall we get a solution of these miseries, then?
If parents select husbands and wives for their children,
then this evil is minimized. The daughters of India
are more practical than sentimental. But very little of
poetry remains in their lives. Again, if people select
their own husbands and wives, that does not seem to
bring much happiness. The Indian woman is generally

very happy; there are not many cases of quarrelling
between husband and wife. On the other hand, in the
United States, where the greatest liberty obtains, the
number of unhappy homes and marriages is large.

Unhappiness is here, there, and everywhere. What
does it show? That, after all, not much happiness has
been gained by all these ideals. We all struggle for
happiness, and as soon as we get a little happiness on
one side, on the other side there comes unhappiness.

Shall we not work to do good, then? Yes, with more
zest than ever. But what this knowledge will do for us
is to break down our fanaticism. The Englishman
will no more be a fanatic and curse the Hindu. He
will learn to respect the customs of different nations.
There will be less of fanaticism and more of real work.
Fanatics cannot work; they waste three-fourths of their
energy. It is the level-headed, calm, practical man who
works. So the power to work will increase from this
idea. Knowing that this is the state of things, we shall
have more patience. The sight of misery or of evil will
not be able to throw us off our balance and make us
run after shadows. Patience will come to us, since we
know that the world will have to go on in its own way.
If, for instance, all men have become good, the animals will have in the meantime evolved into men and
will have to pass through the same state, and so with
the plants.

But one thing is certain: the mighty river is rushing
towards the ocean, and all the drops that constitute
the stream will in time be drawn into that boundless
ocean. So, in this life, with all its miseries and sorrows, its joys and smiles and tears, one thing is certain:

that all things are rushing towards their goal and it is only a question of time when you and I, plants and animals, and every particle of life that exists, must reach the infinite Ocean of Perfection, must attain to Freedom, to God.

Let me repeat once more that the Vedāntic position is neither pessimism nor optimism. It does not say that this world is all evil or all good. It says that our evil is of no less value than our good, and our good of no more value than our evil. They are bound together. This is the world, and knowing this, you work with patience.

What for? Why should we work? If this is the state of things, what shall we do? Why not become agnostics? The modern agnostics also know that there is no solution of this problem, no getting out of this evil of māyā, as we say in our language; therefore they tell us to be satisfied and enjoy life. But here, again, is a mistake, a tremendous mistake, a most illogical mistake. And it is this: What do you mean by life? Do you mean only the life of the senses? In this, every one of us differs only slightly from the brutes. I am sure that no one is present here whose life is only in the senses. Then this present life means something more than that. Our feelings, thoughts, and aspirations are all part and parcel of our life; and is not the struggle towards the great ideal, towards perfection, one of the most important components of what we call life? According to the agnostics we must enjoy life as it is. The agnostic position takes this life, *minus* the ideal of perfection, to be all that exists. That ideal, the agnostic claims, cannot be reached; therefore he must give up the search. But life means, above all, this search after the ideal; the essence of life is going towards perfection. We must have that, and therefore we cannot be agnostics and take the world as it appears.

This nature, this universe, is what is called māyā. All religions are more or less attempts to get beyond nature—the crudest or the most developed, expressed through mythology or symbology, stories of gods or angels or demons, or through stories of saints or seers, great men or prophets, or through the abstractions of philosophy—all have that one object; all are trying to get beyond these limitations. In one word, they are all struggling towards freedom.

Man feels, consciously or unconsciously, that he is bound; he is not what he wants to be. It was taught to him at the very moment he began to look around. That very instant he learnt that he was bound, and he also found that there was something in him which wanted to fly beyond, where the body could not follow, but which was as yet chained down by this limitation. Even in the lowest of religious ideas, where departed ancestors and other spirits, mostly violent and cruel, lurking about the houses of their friends, fond of bloodshed and strong drink, are worshipped—even there we find that one common factor, that of freedom. The man who wants to worship the gods sees in them, above all things, greater freedom than in himself. If a door is closed, he thinks that the gods can get through it, and that walls have no limitations for them. This idea of freedom increases until it comes to the ideal of a Personal God, of which the central concept is that He is a Being beyond the limitations of nature, of māyā.

I see before me, as it were, that in some of the forest retreats this question is being discussed by those ancient sages of India, and that when even the oldest and the holiest among them fail to reach the solution, a young man stands up in the midst of them and declares: "Hear, ye children of immortality! Hear, ye who live in the highest places! I have found the way. By knowing Him who is beyond darkness we can go beyond death."

This māyā is everywhere; it is terrible. Yet we have to work through it. The man who says that he will work when the world has become all good and then he will enjoy bliss is as likely to succeed as the man who sits beside the Ganges and says, "I will ford the river when all the water has run into the ocean." The way is not *with* māyā but *against* it. This is another fact to learn. We are not born as helpers of nature, but as competitors with nature. We are its masters, but we bind ourselves down. Why is this house here? Nature did not build it. Nature says, "Go and live in the forest." Man says, "I will build a house and fight with nature." And he does so. The whole history of humanity is a continuous fight against the so-called laws of nature. And man gains in the end. Coming to the internal world, there too the same fight is going on, the fight between the animal man and the spiritual man, between light and darkness. And here too man becomes victorious. He cuts his way, as it were, out of nature to freedom. We see, then, that beyond this māyā the Vedāntic philosophers find something which is not bound by māyā; and if we can get there, we shall not be bound by māyā. This idea is in some form or other the common property of all religions. But with Vedānta it is only the beginning of religion and not the end. The idea of a Personal God, the Ruler and Creator of this universe, as He has been styled, the Ruler of māyā or nature, is not the end of these Vedāntic ideas; it is only the beginning. The idea grows and grows until the Vedāntist finds that He who, he thought, was standing outside is he himself and is in reality within. He himself is the one who is free, but through limitation he thought he was bound.

MĀYĀ AND THE EVOLUTION OF
THE CONCEPT OF GOD

(Delivered in London, October 20, 1896)

W
E HAVE SEEN that the idea of māyā, which forms, as it were, one of the basic doctrines of Advaita Vedānta, is, in its germ, found even in the Samhitās, and that in reality all the ideas which are developed in the Upanishads are to be found already in the Samhitās in some form or other. Most of you are by this time familiar with the idea of māyā and know that it is sometimes erroneously explained as illusion; and hence when the universe is said to be māyā, it also has to be explained as being illusion. The translation of the word is neither happy nor correct. Māyā is not a theory; it is simply a statement of fact about the universe as it exists; and to understand māyā we must go back to the Samhitās and begin with the conception in the germ.

The Samhitās speak of the devas. These devas were at first understood to be only powerful beings, nothing more. Many of us are horrified when reading the old scriptures, whether of the Greeks, the Hebrews, the Persians, or others, to find that the ancient gods sometimes did things which to us are very repugnant. But when we read these books we entirely forget that we are persons of the nineteenth century and that these gods were beings existing thousands of years ago. We also forget that the people who worshipped these gods

45

found nothing incongruous in their characters, found nothing to frighten them, because they were very much like themselves.

I may also remark that that is the one great lesson we have to learn throughout our lives. In judging others we always judge them by our own ideals. That is not as it should be. Everyone must be judged according to his own ideal, and not by that of anyone else. In our dealings with our fellow beings we constantly labour under this mistake, and I am of opinion that the vast majority of our quarrels with one another arise simply from this one cause: that we are always trying to judge others' gods by our gods, others' ideals by our ideals, and others' motives by our motives. Under certain circumstances I might do a certain thing, and when I see another person taking the same course, I think he has also the same motive actuating him, little dreaming that although the effect may be the same, yet many other causes may produce the same thing. He may have performed the action with quite a different motive from that which impelled me to do it. So in judging of those ancient religions we must not take the standpoint to which we incline, but must put ourselves in the position of the thought and life of those early times.

The idea of the cruel and ruthless Jehovah in the Old Testament has frightened many. But why? What right have they to assume that the Jehovah of the ancient Jews must represent the conventional idea of the God of the present day? And at the same time we must not forget that there will come men after us who will laugh at our ideas of religion and God in the same way that we laugh at those of the ancients. Yet through all these various conceptions runs the golden thread of unity. It is the purpose of Vedānta to discover this thread. "I am the thread that runs through all these various ideas, each one of which is like a pearl," says Lord Krishna. And it is the duty of Vedānta to establish this connecting thread, however incongruous or disgusting may seem these ideas when judged according to the conceptions of today.

These ideas, in the setting of past times, were really not hideous; on the contrary, they were harmonious. It is only when we try to take them out of their setting and apply them to our own present circumstances that the hideousness becomes obvious. For the old surroundings are dead and gone. Just as the ancient Jew has developed into the keen, modern, sharp Jew, and the ancient Āryan into the intellectual Hindu, similarly Jehovah has grown, the devas have grown. The great mistake is in recognizing the evolution of the worshippers, while not acknowledging the evolution of the worshipped. He is not credited with the advance that His devotees have made. The truth is that you and I, as representing ideas, have grown; and these gods too, as representing ideas, have grown.

This may seem somewhat curious to you—that God can grow. He cannot. In the same sense the Real Man never grows. We shall see later on that the Real Man, behind each one of these human manifestations, is immovable, unchangeable, pure, and always perfect. As the tangible man is only an appearance, a partial manifestation of the Real Man, so the idea we form of God is a creation of the mind, only a partial mani-

festation. Behind that is the Real God, who never
changes, the Ever Pure, the Immutable. But the manifestation is always changing, revealing more and more
the Reality behind. When it reveals more of the fact
behind, it is called progression; when it hides more
of the fact behind, it is called retrogression. Thus as
we grow, so the gods grow. From the ordinary point of
view, just as we reveal ourselves, as we evolve, so
the gods reveal themselves.

We shall now be in a position to understand the
theory of māyā. All the religions of the world raise
this question: Why is there disharmony in the universe? Why is there this evil in the universe? We do
not find this question at the very inception of primitive
religious ideas, because the world did not appear incongruous to the primitive man. Circumstances were
not inharmonious for him; there was no clash of opinions; to him there was no antagonism of good and evil.
There was merely a feeling in his own heart of something which said yea and something which said nay.
The primitive man was a man of impulse. He did
what occurred to him; he tried to bring out through
his muscles whatever thought came into his mind. He
never stopped to judge, and seldom tried to check his
impulses. So with the gods: they were also creatures
of impulse. Indra comes and shatters the forces of the
demons. Jehovah is pleased with one person and displeased with another—for what reason, no one knows
or asks; the habit of inquiry had not then arisen, and
whatever He did was regarded as right. There was no
idea of good or evil. The devas did many wicked things
in our sense of the word; again and again Indra and

other gods committed very wicked deeds. But to the worshippers of Indra the ideas of wickedness and evil did not occur; so they did not question them.

With the advance of ethical ideas came the struggle. There arose a certain sense in man, called in different languages and nations by different names. Call it the voice of God, or the result of past education, or whatever else you like, but the effect was that it had a checking power upon the natural impulses of man. There is one impulse in our minds which says, Do. Behind it rises another voice which says, Do not. There is one set of ideas in our minds which is always struggling to get outside through the channels of the senses, and behind that, although it may be thin and weak, there is an infinitely small voice which says, Do not go outside. The two beautiful Sanskrit words for these phenomena are pravritti and nivritti, circling forward and circling inward. It is the circling forward which usually governs our actions. Religion begins with the circling inward. Religion begins with this "Do not." Spirituality begins with this "Do not." When the "Do not" is not there, religion has not begun. And this "Do not" came, causing men's ideas to grow, despite the fighting gods whom they had worshipped.

A little love awoke in the hearts of mankind. It was very small indeed, and even now it is not much greater. It was at first confined to a tribe, embracing perhaps members of the same tribe. These gods loved their tribes and each god was a tribal god, the protector of that tribe. And sometimes the members of a tribe would think of themselves as the descendants of their god, just as the clans in different nations think that they

are the common descendants of the man who was the
founder of the clan. There were in ancient times, and
there are even now, some people who claim to be
descendants not only of these tribal gods, but also of
the sun and the moon. You read in the ancient Sanskrit books of the great heroic emperors of the Solar
and the Lunar Dynasty. They were first worshippers
of the sun and the moon, and gradually came to think
of themselves as descendants of the god of the sun, of
the moon, and so forth. So when these tribal ideas
began to grow, there came a little love, some slight
idea of duty towards each other, a little social organization. Then naturally the idea came: "How can we live
together without bearing and forbearing?" How can
one man live with another without having some time
or other to check his impulses, to restrain himself, to
forbear from doing things which his mind would
prompt him to do? It is impossible. Thus came the
idea of restraint. The whole social fabric is based upon
that idea of restraint, and we all know that the man
or woman who has not learnt the great lesson of bearing and forbearing leads a most miserable life.

Now, when these ideas of religion came, a glimpse
of something higher, more ethical, dawned upon the
intellect of mankind. The old gods were found to be
incongruous—those boisterous, fighting, drinking, beef-
eating gods of the ancients, whose delight was in the
smell of burning flesh and libations of strong liquor.
Sometimes Indra drank so much that he fell upon the
ground and talked unintelligibly. These gods could no
longer be tolerated. The notion had arisen of inquiring
into motives, and the gods had to come in for their share

of inquiry. The reason for such and such actions was demanded, and the reason was wanting. Therefore men gave up these gods, or rather they developed higher ideas concerning them. They took a survey, as it were, of all the actions and qualities of the gods and discarded those which they could not harmonize, and kept those which they could understand, and combined them, labelling them with one name, Deva-deva, the God of gods. The God to be worshipped was no more a simple symbol of power; something more was required than that. He was an ethical God; He loved mankind and did good to mankind. But the idea of God still remained. They increased His ethical significance and increased also His power. He became the most ethical Being in the universe, as well as almost almighty.

But all this patchwork would not do. As the explanation assumed greater proportions, the difficulty it sought to solve did the same. If the virtues of God increased in arithmetical progression, the difficulty and doubt increased in geometrical progression. The difficulty about Jehovah was very little beside the difficulty about the God of the universe. And this question remains to the present day: Why, under the reign of an almighty and all-loving God of the universe, should diabolical things be allowed to remain? Why so much more misery than happiness and so much more wickedness than good?

We may shut our eyes to all these things, but the fact still remains that this world is a hideous world. At best it is the hell of Tantalus. Here we are, with strong impulses and stronger cravings for sense enjoy-

ments, but cannot satisfy them. There rises a wave
which impels us forward in spite of our own will, and
as soon as we move one step there comes a blow. We
are all doomed to live here like Tantalus. Further,
ideals come into our heads far beyond the limit of our
sense ideals, but when we seek to express them we
cannot do so. On the contrary, we are crushed by the
surging mass around us. Yet if I give up all idealism
and lead a worldly life, my existence becomes that
of a brute, and I debase and degrade myself. Neither
way is happiness. Unhappiness is the fate of those
who are content to live in this world as they are. A
thousand times greater misery is the fate of those who
dare to stand forth for truth and for higher things,
and who dare to ask for something higher than mere
brute existence here.

These are facts; but there is no explanation. There
cannot be any explanation. But Vedānta shows the
way out. You must bear in mind that I have to tell
you facts that will frighten you sometimes; but if you
remember what I say, think of it, and digest it, it
will be yours, it will raise you higher and make you
capable of understanding and of living in truth.

Now, it is a fact that this world is a Tantalus' hell.
We do not know anything about this universe; yet at
the same time we cannot say that we do not know.
I cannot assert that this universe exists: when I think,
I realize that I do not know anything about it. It may
be an entire delusion of my brain. I may be dreaming
all the time: I am dreaming that I am talking to you
and that you are listening to me. No one can prove that
it is not a dream. My brain itself may be a dream;

and as to that, no one has ever seen his own brain. We all take it for granted. My own body, too, I take for granted. So it is with everything. At the same time I cannot say that I do not know.

This standing between knowledge and ignorance, in this mysterious twilight, the mingling of truth and falsehood—and where they meet, no one knows—is the fate of every one of us. We are walking in the midst of a dream, half sleeping, half waking, passing all our lives in a haze. This is the fate of all sense knowledge. This is the fate of all philosophy, of all our boasted science, of all our boasted human knowledge. This is the universe.

Whether we speak of matter or spirit or mind or anything else, the fact remains the same: we cannot say that they are; we cannot say that they are not. We cannot say that they are one; we cannot say that they are many. This eternal play of light and darkness —indiscriminate, indistinguishable, inseparable—is always there. Because of it the universe appears real, yet at the same time not real, and we appear awake, yet at the same time asleep. This is a statement of fact, and this is what is called māyā.

We are born in this māyā, we live in it, we think in it, we dream in it. We are philosophers in it, we are spiritual men in it, nay, we are devils in this māyā and we are gods in this māyā. Stretch your ideas as far as you can, take them higher and higher, call them infinite or by any other name you please—even these ideas are within māyā. It cannot be otherwise. The whole of human knowledge is a generalization of this māyā, an attempt to know it as it appears to be.

This is the work of nāma-rupa, name and form. Everything that has form, everything that calls up an idea
in your mind, is within māyā; for everything that is
bound by the laws of time, space, and causation is
within māyā.

Let us go back a little to those early ideas of God
and see what became of them. We perceive at once
that the idea of some Being who is eternally loving
us, eternally unselfish and almighty, ruling this universe, cannot satisfy men. "What sort of just, merciful
God is this?" asks the philosopher. Does He not see
millions and millions of His children perish, in the
form of men and animals; for who can live one
moment here without killing others? Can you draw a
breath without destroying thousands of lives? You live
because millions die. Every moment of your life, every
breath that you breathe, is death to thousands; every
movement that you make is death to millions. Every
morsel that you eat is death to millions. Why should
they die?

There is an old sophism, that they are very low
existences. Suppose they are—which is questionable,
for who knows whether the ant is greater than the
man, or the man than the ant? Who can prove it one
way or the other? Apart from that question, even
taking it for granted that these are very low beings,
still why should they die? If they are low they have
more reason to live. Why not? Because they live more
in the senses, they feel pleasure and pain a thousand-
fold more than you or I can do. Which of us eats a
dinner with the same gusto as a dog or a wolf? None,
because our energies are not in the senses; they are

in the intellect, in the spirit. But in animals the whole soul is in the senses; they become mad after sense pleasure, and enjoy things with an intensity which we human beings never dream of; and the pain is commensurate with the pleasure. Pleasure and pain are meted out in equal measure. If the pleasure felt by animals is so much keener than that felt by man, it follows that the animals' sense of pain is as keen, if not keener, than man's. So the fact is that the pain and misery men feel in dying is intensified a thousand-fold in animals, and yet we kill them without troubling about their misery. This is māyā.

If we suppose there is a Personal God like a human being, who made everything, these so-called explanations and theories which try to prove that out of evil comes good are not sufficient. Let twenty thousand good things come, but why should they come from evil? On that principle I might cut the throats of others because I want the full pleasure of my five senses. That is no reason. Why should good come through evil? The question remains to be answered, and it cannot be answered. The philosophy of India was compelled to admit this.

Vedānta was—and is—the boldest system of religion. It stopped nowhere, and it had one advantage: There was no body of priests who sought to suppress men who tried to tell the truth. There was always absolute religious freedom. In India the bondage of superstition is a social one; here in the West society is very free. Social matters in India are very strict, but religious opinion is free. In England a man may dress any way he likes or eat with anyone he likes—no one

objects; but if he misses attending church, then Mrs.
Grundy is down on him. He has to conform first to
what society says on religion, and then he may think
of the truth. In India, on the other hand, if a man
dines with one who does not belong to his own caste,
down comes society with all its terrible power and
crushes him then and there. If he wants to dress a
little differently from the way in which his ancestors
dressed ages ago, he is done for. I have heard of a
man who was cast out by society because he went several miles to see the first railway train. Well, we shall
presume that that was not true. But in religion we
find atheists, materialists, and Buddhists, creeds, opinions, and speculations of every phase and variety, some
of a most startling character, living side by side.
Preachers of all sects go about teaching and getting
adherents, and at the very gates of the temples of gods,
the brāhmins—to their credit be it said—allow even
materialists to stand and give forth their opinions.

Buddha died at a ripe old age. I remember a friend
of mine, a great American scientist, who was fond of
reading his life. He did not like the death of Buddha,
because he was not crucified. What a false idea! For
a man to be great he must be murdered! Such ideas
never prevailed in India. This great Buddha travelled
all over India, denouncing her gods, and even the
God of the universe, and yet he lived to a good old
age. For eighty years he lived, and he converted half
the country.

Then there were the Chārvākas, who preached horrible things, the most rank, undisguised materialism,
such as in the nineteenth century they dare not openly

preach. These Chārvākas were allowed to preach, from temple to temple and city to city, that religion was all nonsense, that it was priestcraft, that the Vedas were the words and writings of fools, rogues, and demons, and that there was neither God nor an eternal soul. If there was a soul, why did it not come back after death, drawn by the love of wife and child? Their idea was that if there was a soul it must still love after death and want good things to eat and nice dress. Yet no one hurt these Chārvākas.

You must remember that freedom is the first condition of growth. We in India allowed liberty in spiritual matters, and we have a tremendous power in the realm of religion even today. You grant the same liberty in social matters, and so have a splendid social organization. We have not given any freedom in the expansion of social matters, and ours is a cramped society. You have never given any freedom in religious matters, but with fire and sword have enforced your beliefs; and the result is that religion is a stunted, degenerated growth in the European mind. In India we have to take off the shackles from society; in Europe the chains must be taken from the feet of spiritual progress. Then will come a wonderful growth and development of man. If we discover that there is a unity running through all these developments, spiritual, moral, and social, we shall find that religion, in the fullest sense of the word, must come into society and into our every-day life. In the light of Vedānta you will understand that all sciences are but manifestations of religion, and so is everything that exists in this world.

In society we find two sets of opinions, the one

denunciatory and the other positive and constructive.
It is a most curious fact that in every society you find
them. Suppose there is an evil in society: you will
find immediately one group rising up and denouncing
it in vindictive fashion; and this sometimes degenerates into fanaticism. There are fanatics in every
society, and women frequently join in these outcries,
because of their impulsive nature. Every fanatic who
gets up and denounces something can secure a following. It is very easy to break down; a maniac can break
anything he likes, but it would be hard for him to
build up anything. These fanatics may do some good,
according to their lights, but they do much more harm.
Social institutions are not made in a day, and to change
them means removing the cause. Suppose there is an
evil: denouncing it will not remove it, but you must
go to work at the root. First find out the cause, then
remove it, and the effect will be removed also. Mere
outcry will not produce any result, unless indeed it
produces misfortune.

There are others who have sympathy in their hearts
and who understand the idea that we must go deep
into the cause. These are the great saints. One fact
you must remember: all the great teachers of the world
have declared that they came not to destroy but to
fulfil. Many times this has not been understood, and
their forbearance has been thought to be an unworthy
compromise with existing popular opinions. Even now
you occasionally hear that these prophets and great
teachers were rather cowardly and dared not say and
do what they thought was right. But that is not so.
Fanatics little understand the infinite power of love

in the hearts of these great sages, who looked upon the inhabitants of this world as their children. They were the real fathers, the real gods, filled with infinite sympathy and patience for everyone; they were ready to bear and forbear. They knew how human society should grow, and patiently, slowly, surely, went on applying their remedies, not by denouncing and frightening people, but by gently and kindly leading them upwards, step by step. Such were the writers of the Upanishads. They knew full well that the old ideas of God were not reconcilable with the advanced ethical ideas of the time; they knew full well that what the atheists were preaching contained a good deal of truth, nay, great nuggets of truth; but at the same time they understood that those who wished to sever the thread that bound the beads, who wanted to build a new society in the air, would entirely fail.

We never build anew; we simply rearrange. We cannot have anything new; we only change the position of things. The seed grows into the tree patiently and gently. We must direct our energies towards the truth, and fulfil the truth that exists, not try to make new truths. Thus, instead of denouncing these old ideas of God as unfit for modern times, the ancient sages began to seek out the reality that was in them. The result was the Vedānta philosophy. From the old deities and from the monotheistic God, the Ruler of the universe, they ascended to yet higher and higher ideas. And the highest of them all they called the Impersonal Absolute, in which they beheld the oneness of the universe.

He who sees in this world of manifoldness that One

running through all; in this world of death, he who finds that one infinite Life; and in this world of insentience and ignorance, he who finds that one Light and Knowledge—unto him belongs eternal peace, unto none else, unto none else.

MĀYĀ AND FREEDOM

(Delivered in London, October 22, 1896)

"TRAILING CLOUDS of glory do we come," says the poet. Not all of us come trailing clouds of glory, however; some of us come trailing black fogs. There can be no question about that. But every one of us comes into this world to fight, as on a battlefield. We come here weeping, to fight our way as well as we can and to make a path for ourselves through this infinite ocean of life. Forward we go, having long ages behind us and an immense expanse beyond. So on we go, till death comes and takes us off the field—victorious or defeated, we do not know. And this is māyā.

Hope is dominant in the heart of childhood. The whole world is a golden vision to the opening eyes of the child; he thinks his will is supreme. As he moves onward, at every step nature stands as an adamantine wall, barring his farther progress. He may hurl himself against it again and again, striving to break through. The farther he goes, the farther recedes the ideal, till death comes and there is release, perhaps. And this is māyā.

A man of science rises. He is thirsting after knowledge. No sacrifice is too great, no struggle too hopeless for him. He moves onward, discovering secret after secret of nature, searching out the secrets from its innermost heart—and what for? What is it all for? Why should we give him glory? Why should he acquire

61

fame? Does not nature do infinitely more than any human being can do? And nature is dull, insentient. Why should it be glorious to imitate the dull, the insentient? Nature can hurl a thunderbolt of any magnitude to any distance. If a man can do one small part as much, we praise him and laud him to the skies. Why? Why should we praise him for imitating nature, imitating death, imitating dullness, imitating insentience? The force of gravitation can pull to pieces the biggest mass that ever existed; yet it is insentient. What glory is there in imitating the insentient? Yet we are all struggling after that. And this is māyā.

The senses drag the human soul out. Man is seeking for pleasure and for happiness where it can never be found. For countless ages we have been taught that this search is futile and vain; there is no happiness here. But we cannot learn; it is impossible for us to do so except through our own experiences. We try them, and a blow comes. Do we learn then? Not even then. Like moths hurling themselves against the flame, we hurl ourselves again and again into sense pleasures, hoping to find satisfaction there. We return again and again with freshened energy; thus we go on till, crippled and cheated, we die. And this is māyā.

So with our intellect. In our desire to solve the mysteries of the universe, we cannot stop our questioning; we feel we must know and cannot believe that no knowledge is ever gained. A few steps, and there arises the wall of beginningless and endless time which we cannot surmount. A few steps, and there appears a wall of boundless space which cannot be surmounted, and the whole is irrevocably bound in by the walls of cause and effect. We cannot go beyond them. Yet we struggle, and still have to struggle. And this is māyā.

With every breath, with every pulsation of the heart, with every one of our movements, we think we are free, and the very same moment we are shown that we are not: we are born slaves, nature's bond-slaves, in body, in mind, in all our thoughts, in all our feelings. And this is māyā.

There is never a mother who does not think her child is a born genius, the most extraordinary child that was ever born. She dotes upon her child. Her whole soul is in the child. The child grows up, perhaps becomes a drunkard, a brute, and ill-treats the mother; and the more he ill-treats her, the more her love increases. The world lauds it as the unselfish love of the mother, little dreaming that the mother is a slave; she cannot help herself. She would a thousand times rather throw off the burden, but she cannot. So she covers it with a mass of flowers, which she calls wonderful love. And this is māyā.

We are all like this in the world. A legend tells how once Nārada said to Krishna, "Lord, show me māyā." A few days passed, and Krishna asked Nārada to make a trip with Him towards a forest. After walking several miles Krishna said, "Nārada, I am thirsty; can you fetch some water for Me?" "I will go at once, Sir, and get you water." So Nārada went. At a little distance there was a village. He entered the village in search of water and knocked at a door, which was opened by a most beautiful young girl. At the sight of her he immediately forgot that his Master was waiting for water, perhaps dying for want of it. He forgot everything and began to talk with the girl. Gradually that talk ripened into love. He asked the father for his daughter, and they were married and lived there and had children. Thus twelve years passed. His father-in-law died; he inherited his property. He lived, as he seemed to think, a very happy life with his wife and children, his fields and his cattle, and so forth. Then came a flood. One night the river rose until it over-flowed its banks and flooded the whole village. Houses fell, men and animals were swept away and drowned, and everything was floating in the rush of the stream. Nārada had to escape. With one hand he held his wife, and with the other, two of his children; another child was on his shoulders, and he was trying to ford this tremendous flood. After a few steps he found the current was too strong, and the child on his shoulders fell and was borne away. A cry of despair came from Nārada. In trying to save that child, he lost his grasp upon the others, and they also were lost. At last his wife, whom he clasped with all his might, was torn away by the current, and he was thrown on the bank, weeping and wailing in bitter lamentation. Behind him there came a gentle voice: "My child, where is the water? You went to fetch a pitcher of water, and I am waiting for you. You have been gone for quite half an hour." "Half an hour!" Nārada exclaimed. Twelve whole years had passed through his mind, and all these scenes had happened in half an hour! And this is māyā. In one form or another we are all in it. It is a most difficult and intricate state of things to un-derstand. It has been preached in every country, taught everywhere, but only believed in by a few, because until we get the experiences ourselves we cannot believe in it. What does it show? Something very terrible: that it is all futile.

Time, the all-destroyer, comes, and nothing is left. He swallows up the saint and the sinner, the king and the peasant, the beautiful and the ugly; he leaves nothing. Everything is rushing towards that one goal: destruction. Our knowledge, our arts, our sciences— everything is rushing towards it. None can stem the tide, none can hold it back for a minute. We may try to forget it, in the same way that persons in a plague-stricken city try to create oblivion by drinking, dancing, and other vain attempts, and so becoming paralysed. So we are trying to forget, trying to create oblivion by all sorts of sense pleasures. And this is māyā.

Two solutions have been proposed. One, which everyone knows, is very common, and that is: "It is all very true, but do not think of it. 'Make hay while the sun shines,' as the proverb says. It is true that there is suffering; but do not mind it. Seize the few pleasures you can, do what little you can, do not look at the dark side of the picture, but always towards the hopeful, the positive side." There is some truth in this, but there is also a danger. The truth is that it is a good motive power; hope and a positive ideal are very good motive powers for our lives. But there is a certain danger in them. The danger lies in our giving up the struggle in despair, as do those who preach: "Take the world as it is; sit down as calmly and comfortably as you can, and be contented with all these miseries. When you receive blows, say they are not blows but flowers; and when you are driven about like slaves, say that you are free. Day and night tell lies to others and to your own souls, because that is the only way to live happily."

This is what is called practical wisdom, and never was it more prevalent in the world than in this nineteenth century, because never were harder blows hit than at the present time, never was competition keener, never were men so cruel to their fellow men as now; and therefore this consolation must be offered. It is put forward in the strongest way at the present time; but it fails, as it always must fail. We cannot hide carrion with roses; it is impossible. It would not avail long; for soon the roses would fade and the carrion would be worse than before. So with our lives. We may try to cover our old and festering sore with cloth of gold, but there comes a day when the cloth of gold is removed and the sore in all its ugliness is revealed.

Is there no hope, then? True it is that we are all slaves of māyā, are all born in māyā and live in māyā. Is there then no way out, no hope? That we are all miserable, that this world is really a prison, that even our so-called "trailing glory" is but a prison-house, and that even our intellects and minds are prison-houses, has been known for ages upon ages. There has never been a man, there has never been a human soul, who has not felt this some time or other, however he may talk. And the old people feel it most, because in them is the accumulated experience of a whole life, because they cannot be easily cheated by the lies of nature. Is there no way out?

We find that with all this, with this terrible fact

before us, in the midst of sorrow and suffering, even
in this world where life and death are synonymous,
even here a still, small voice has been ringing through
all the ages, in every country, and in every heart:
"This My māyā is divine, made up of the gunas, and
very difficult to cross. Yet those that come unto Me
cross the river of māyā." "Come unto Me, all ye that
labour and are heavy laden, and I will give you rest."
This is the voice that is leading us forward. Man has
heard it—and is hearing it—all through the ages. This
voice comes to man when everything seems to be lost,
and hope has fled, when man's dependence on his own
strength has been crushed down, and everything seems
to melt away between his fingers, and life is a hopeless
ruin. Then he hears it. This is called religion.

On the one side, therefore, is the bold assertion that
this is all nonsense, that this is māyā; but along with
it there is the hopeful assertion that from this māyā
there is a way out. On the other hand, practical men
tell us: "Don't bother your heads about such nonsense
as religion and metaphysics. Live here; this is a very
bad world, indeed, but make the best of it." Which,
put in plain language, means: Live a hypocritical,
lying life, a life of continuous fraud, covering your old
sores in the best way you can; go on putting patch
after patch, until everything is lost and you are a mass
of patchwork. This is what is called practical wisdom.
Those who are satisfied with this patchwork will never
come to religion.

Religion begins with a tremendous dissatisfaction
with the present state of things, with our lives, and a
hatred, an intense hatred, for this patching up of life,

an unbounded disgust for fraud and lies. He alone can be religious who dares to say what the mighty Buddha once said under the Bo-tree, when this idea of practicality appeared before him and he saw that it was nonsense, and yet could not find a way out. When the temptation came to him to give up his search after truth, to go back to the world and live the old life of fraud, calling things by wrong names, telling lies to himself and to everybody, he, the giant, conquered it and said: "Death is better than a vegetating ignorant life; it is better to die on the battlefield than to live a life of defeat." This is the basis of religion.

When a man takes this stand he is on the way to find the truth, he is on the way to God. That determination must be the first impulse towards becoming religious. I will hew out a way for myself. I will know the truth or give up my life in the attempt. For on this side it is nothing, it is gone, it is vanishing every day. The beautiful, hopeful young person of today is the veteran of tomorrow. Hopes and joys and pleasures will die like blossoms with tomorow's frost. That is one side. On the other, there are the great charms of conquest, victories over all the ills of life, victories over life itself, the conquest of the universe. On that side men can stand. Those who dare, therefore, to struggle for victory, for truth, for religion, are on the right path, and that is what the Vedas preach. "Be not in despair; the way is very difficult, like walking on the blade of a razor. Yet despair not; arise, awake, and find the ideal, the goal."

Now, all these various manifestations of religion, in whatever shape or form they have come to mankind,

have one common, central basis. It is the preaching
of freedom, the way out of this world. They never
came to reconcile the world and religion, but to cut
the Gordian knot, to establish religion in its own ·
ideal, and not to compromise with the world. That
is what every religion preaches; and the duty of
Vedānta is to harmonize all these aspirations, to make
manifest the common ground between all the religions
of the world, the highest as well as the lowest. What
we call the most arrant superstition and the highest
philosophy really have a common aim, in that they
both try to show the way out of the same difficulty;
and in most cases this way is through the help of
someone who is not himself bound by the laws of
nature, in one word, someone who is free. In spite
of all the difficulties and differences of opinion about
the nature of the one free agent, whether he is a
Personal God or a sentient being like man, whether
masculine, feminine, or neuter—and the discussions
have been endless—the fundamental idea is the same.
In spite of the almost hopeless contradictions of the
different systems, we find the golden thread of unity
running through them all; and in this philosophy, this
golden thread has been traced, revealed little by little
to our view; and the first step to this revelation is the
knowledge that we are all advancing towards freedom.

One curious fact present in the midst of all our
joys and sorrows, difficulties and struggles, is that we
are surely journeying towards freedom. The question
raised was this: "What is this universe? From what
does it arise? Into what does it go?" And the answer
was: "In freedom it rises, in freedom it rests, and into

freedom it melts away." This idea of freedom, you cannot relinquish; your actions, your very lives, will be lost without it. Every moment nature is proving us to be slaves and not free. Yet simultaneously rises the other idea, that still we are free. At every step we are knocked down, as it were, by māyā, and shown that we are bound; and yet at the same moment, together with this blow, together with this feeling that we are bound, comes the other feeling that we are free. Some inner voice tells us that we are free. But if we attempt to realize that freedom, to make it manifest, we find the difficulties almost insuperable. Yet in spite of that, it insists on asserting itself inwardly: "I am free, I am free." And if you study all the various religions of the world you will find this idea expressed.

Not only religion—you must not take this word in its narrow sense—but the whole life of society, is the assertion of that one principle of freedom. All movements are the assertion of that one freedom. That voice has been heard by everyone, whether he knows it or not, that voice which declares, "Come unto Me, all ye that labour and are heavy laden." It may not be in the same language, or the same form of speech, but in some form or other that voice calling for freedom has been with us. Yes, we are born here on account of that voice; every one of our movements is towards that end. We are all rushing towards freedom, we are all following that voice, whether we know it or not; as the children of the village were attracted by the music of the flute-player, so we are all following the music of the voice without knowing it.

We are ethical when we follow that voice. Not only

the human soul, but all creatures from the lowest
to the highest have heard the voice and are rushing
towards it, and in the struggle are either combining
with each other or pushing each other out of the way.
Thus come competition, joys, struggles, life, pleasure,
and death; and the whole universe is nothing but the
result of this mad struggle to reach the voice. This is
the manifestation of nature.

What happens then? The scene begins to shift. As
soon as you know the voice and understand what it is,
the whole scene changes. The same world which was
the ghastly battlefield of māyā is now changed into
something good and beautiful. We no longer curse
nature or say that the world is horrible and that it is
all vain; we need no longer weep and wail. As soon
as we understand the voice, we see the reason why this
struggle should be here—this fight, this competition,
these difficulties, this cruelty, these little pleasures
and joys; we see that they are in the nature of things,
because without them there would be no going towards
the voice, which we are destined to attain, whether
we know it or not. All human life, all nature, therefore, is struggling to attain to freedom. The sun is
moving towards the goal; so is the earth in circling
round the sun; so is the moon in circling round the
earth. To that goal the planets are moving and the air
is blowing. Everything is struggling towards that. The
saint is going towards that voice; he cannot help it;
it is no glory to him. So is the sinner. The charitable
man is going straight towards that voice, and cannot be hindered. The miser is also going towards the
same destination. The greatest worker of good hears

the same voice within; he cannot resist it; he must go
towards the voice. So is the most arrant idler. One
stumbles more than another; him who stumbles more
we call bad, and him who stumbles less we call good.
Good and bad are never two different things; they
are one and the same. The difference is not one of
kind, but of degree.

Now, if the manifestation of this power of freedom
really governs the whole universe, applying that fact
to religion, we find that this idea has been the one
assertion of religion throughout. Take the lowest form
of religion, where there is the worship of departed
ancestors or certain powerful and cruel gods; what
is the prominent idea about the gods or ancestors? It
is that they are superior to nature, not bound by its
restrictions. The worshipper has, no doubt, very
limited control of nature. He himself cannot pass
through a wall or fly up into the skies, but the gods
whom he worships can do these things. What is
meant by that, philosophically? That the assertion of
freedom is there, that the gods whom he worships
are superior to nature as he knows it. So with those
who worship still higher beings. As the idea of nature
expands, the idea of the soul which is superior to
nature also expands, until we come to what we call
monotheism, which holds that there is māyā, or nature,
and that there is some Being who is the Ruler of this
māyā.

Here Vedānta begins, where these monotheistic
ideas first appear. But the Vedānta philosophy wants
further explanation. This explanation that there is
a Being beyond all these manifestations of māyā, who

is superior to and independent of māyā and who is attracting us towards Himself, and that we are all going towards Him, is very good, says Vedānta; but yet the perception is not clear, the vision is dim and hazy, although it does not directly contradict reason.

One of your hymns says, "Nearer my God to Thee." The same hymn would be very good to the Vedāntist, only he would change a word and make it "Nearer my God to Me." The idea that the goal is far off, far beyond nature, attracting us all towards it, has to be changed; the goal has to be brought nearer and nearer, without degrading or debasing it. The God of heaven becomes the God in nature, and the God in nature becomes the God who is nature, and the God who is nature becomes the God within this temple of the body, and the God dwelling in the temple of the body at last becomes the temple itself, becomes the soul and man—and there Vedānta reaches the last words it can teach. He whom the sages have been seeking in all these places is in our own hearts; the voice that you heard was right, says Vedānta, but the direction you gave to the voice was wrong. The ideal of freedom that you perceived was correct, but you projected it outside yourself, and that was your mistake. Bring it nearer and nearer, until you find that it was all the time within you, it was the Self of your own self. That freedom was your own nature, and this māyā never bound you.

Nature never had power over you. Like a frightened child you were dreaming that it was throttling you. The release from this fear is the goal: not only to see it intellectually, but to perceive it, actualize it,

much more definitely than we perceive this world.
Then we shall know that we are free. Then, and
then alone, will all difficulties vanish, then will all
the perplexities of the heart be smoothed away, all
crookedness be made straight; then will vanish the
delusion of manifoldness and nature. Māyā, instead
of being a horrible, hopeless dream, as it is now, will
become beautiful; this earth, instead of being a prison-
house, will become our playground; and even dangers
and difficulties, even all sufferings, will become deified
and show us their real nature, will show us that behind
everything, as the substance of everything, He is standing, and that He is our own real Self.

GOD IN EVERYTHING

(Delivered in London, October 27, 1896)

WE ARE AWARE that the greater portion of our life must of necessity be filled with evil, however we may resist it, and that this mass of evil is practically infinite for us. We have been struggling to remedy this since the beginning of time; yet everything remains very much the same. The more we discover remedies, the more we find ourselves beset by subtler evils. We have also seen that all religions propose a God as the one way of escaping these difficulties. All religions tell us that if we take the world as it is, as most practical people would advise us to do in this age, then nothing will be left to us but evil. They further assert that there is something beyond this world. This life of the five senses, life in the material world, is not all; it is only a small portion, and merely superficial. Behind and beyond is the Infinite, in which there is no more evil. Some people call It God, some Allah, some Jehovah, Jove, and so on. The Vedāntist calls It Brahman.

The first impression we get of the advice given by religion is that we had better terminate our existence. To the question as to how to cure the evils of life, the answer apparently is, Give up life. It reminds one of an old story. A mosquito settled on the head of a man, and a friend, wishing to kill the mosquito, gave it such a blow that he killed both man and mosquito.

The remedy for evil seems to suggest a similar course of action. Life is indeed full of ills; the world is full of evil. That is a fact no one who is old enough to know the world can deny. But what is the remedy proposed by all the religions? That this world is nothing; beyond this world is something which is very real. Here comes the difficulty. The remedy seems to destroy everything. How can that be a remedy? Is there no way out, then?

Vedānta says that what all the religions declare is perfectly true, but it should be properly understood. Often it is misunderstood, because the religions are not very clear in their meaning. What we really want is head and heart combined. The heart is great indeed; it is through the heart that the great inspirations of life come. I would a hundred times rather have a little heart and no brains than be all brains and no heart. Life is possible, progress is possible, for him who has a heart; but he who has no heart and only brains dies of dryness. At the same time we know that he who is carried away by his heart alone has to undergo many ills; for now and then he is liable to tumble into pitfalls. The combination of heart and head is what we want. I do not mean that a man should compromise his heart for his brains or vice versa; but let everyone have an infinite amount of heart and feeling, and at the same time an infinite amount of reason. Is there any limit to what we want in this world? Is not the world infinite? There is room for an infinite amount of feeling, and so also for an infinite amount of knowledge and reason. Let them come together without limit; let them run together, as it were, parallel with each other.

Most of the religions understand this fact, but the error into which they all seem to fall is the same: they are carried away by the heart, the feelings. There is evil in the world; give up the world—that is the great teaching, and the only teaching, no doubt. Give up the world. There cannot be two opinions: to understand the truth every one of us has to give up error. There cannot be two opinions: every one of us, in order to be good, must give up evil. There cannot be two opinions: every one of us, to have life, must give up what is death. And yet, what remains to us if this theory involves giving up the life of the senses, life as we know it? And what else do we mean by life? If we give this up, what remains?

We shall understand this better when, later on, we come to the more philosophical portions of Vedānta. But for the present I beg to state that in Vedānta alone we find a rational solution of the problem. Here I can only lay before you what Vedānta seeks to teach; and that is the deification of the world.

Vedānta does not in reality denounce the world. The ideal of renunciation nowhere attains such a height as in the teachings of Vedānta; but at the same time, no dry suicidal advice is intended. It really means deification of the world: giving up the world as we think of it, as we know it, as it appears to us. Knowing what it really is, deify it; it is God alone.

We read at the commencement of one of the oldest of the Upanishads: "Whatever exists in this universe is to be covered with the Lord." We have to cover

everything with the Lord Himself, not by a false sort
of optimism, not by blinding our eyes to evil, but by
really seeing God in everything. Thus we have to
give up the world. And when the world is given up,
what remains? God. What is meant? You can have
your wife; you certainly do not have to abandon her;
but you are to see God in your wife. Give up your
children—what does that mean? To turn them out of
doors, as some human brutes do in every country?
Certainly not. That is diabolism; it is not religion.
But see God in your children. So in everything. In
life and in death, in happiness and in misery, the
Lord is equally present. The whole world is full of
the Lord. Open your eyes and see Him.

This is what Vedānta teaches: Give up the world
which you have conjectured, because your conjecture
was based upon a very partial experience, upon very
poor reasoning, and upon your own weaknesses. Give
it up. The world we have been thinking of so long,
the world we have been clinging to so long, is a false
world of our own creation. Give that up. Open your
eyes and see that, as such, it never existed; it was a
dream, māyā. What existed was the Lord Himself. It
is He who is in the child, in the wife, and in the
husband; it is He who is in the good and in the bad.
He is in the sin and in the sinner; He is in life and
in death.

A tremendous assertion indeed! Yet that is the
theme which Vedānta wants to demonstrate, to teach,
and to preach. This is just the opening theme.

We avoid the dangers of life and its evils by seeing
God in everything. Do not desire anything. What

makes us miserable? The cause of all the miseries from which we suffer is desire. You desire something, and the desire is not fulfilled; the result is distress. If there is no desire, there is no suffering. But here, too, there is the danger of my being misunderstood. So it is necessary to explain what I mean by giving up desire and becoming free from all misery. The walls have no desires and they never suffer. True, but they never evolve. This chair has no desires; it never suffers; but it is always a chair. There is a glory in happiness; there is a glory in suffering. If I may say so, there is a utility in evil too. The great lesson in misery we all know. There are hundreds of things we have done in our lives which we wish we had never done, but which, at the same time, have been great teachers. As for me, I am glad I have done something good and many things bad; glad I have done something right, and glad I have committed many errors; because every one of them has been a great lesson. I, as I am now, am the resultant of all I have done, all I have thought. Every action and thought have had their effect, and these effects are the sum total of my progress.

We all understand that desires are wrong; but what is meant by giving up desires? How could life go on? It would be the same suicidal advice, killing the desire and the man too. The solution is this: not that you should not have property, not that you should not have things which are necessary and even things which are luxuries—have all that you want, and more; only know the truth about property: that it does not belong to anybody. Have no idea of proprietorship, possession. You are not anybody, nor am I anybody, nor is anyone else. All belong to the Lord. The opening verse of the *Iśa Upanishad* tells us to cover everything with the Lord. God is in the wealth that you enjoy. He is in the desire that rises in your mind. He is in the things you buy to satisfy your desire; He is in your beautiful attire, in your beautiful ornaments. This is the line of thought. All will be metamorphosed as soon as you begin to see things in that light. If you put God in your every movement, in your conversation, in your form, in everything, the whole scene will change, and the world, instead of appearing as one of woe and misery, will become a heaven.

"The kingdom of heaven is within you," says Jesus. So says Vedānta and every great teacher. "He that hath eyes to see, let him see, and he that hath ears to hear, let him hear." Vedānta proves that the truth for which we have been searching all this time is present now and was all the time with us. In our ignorance we thought we had lost it, and went about the world crying and weeping, struggling to find the truth, while all along it was dwelling in our own hearts. There alone can we find it.

If we understand the giving up of the world in its old, crude sense, then it would come to this: that we must not work—that we must be idle, sitting like lumps of earth, neither thinking nor doing anything—but must become fatalists, driven about by every circumstance, ordered about by the laws of nature, drifting from place to place. That would be the result. But that is not what is meant. We must work. Ordinary men work, driven by false desires—what do they know of work? If a man is impelled by his impulses, desires, and senses, what does he know about work? He works who is not impelled by his own desires, by any selfishness whatsoever. He works who has no ulterior motive in view. He works who has nothing to gain from work.

Who enjoys a picture—the seller or the seer? The seller is busy with his accounts, computing what his gain will be, how much profit he will realize from the picture. His brain is full of that. He is looking at the hammer and watching the bids. He is intent on hearing how fast the bids are rising. That man is enjoying the picture who has gone there without any intention of buying or selling. He looks at the picture and enjoys it. So this whole universe is a picture, and when these desires have vanished, men will enjoy the world; then this buying and selling and these foolish ideas of possession will be ended. The money-lender gone, the buyer gone, the seller gone, this world remains a picture, a beautiful painting.

I have never read of any more beautiful conception of God than the following: "He is the Great Poet, the Ancient Poet. The whole universe is His poem, coming in verses and rhymes and rhythms, written in Infinite Bliss." When we have given up desires, then alone shall we be able to read and enjoy this universe of God. Then everything will become deified. Nooks and corners, by-ways and shady places, which we thought dark and unholy, will all be deified. They will all reveal their true nature, and we shall smile at ourselves and think that all this weeping and crying has been but child's-play, and that we were only standing by, watching.

So do your work, says Vedānta. And it advises us
how to work: by giving up—giving up the apparent,
illusive world. What is meant by that? Seeing God
everywhere. Thus do your work. Desire to live a
hundred years; have all earthly desires, if you wish,
only deify them, convert them into heaven. Have the
desire to live a long life of helpfulness, of blissfulness
and activity, on this earth. Thus working, you will
find the way out. There is no other way. If a man
plunges headlong into the foolish luxuries of the world
without knowing the truth, he has missed his footing;
he cannot reach the goal. And if a man curses the
world, goes into a forest, mortifies his flesh, and kills
himself little by little by starvation, makes his heart
a barren waste, kills out all feeling, and becomes harsh,
stern, and dried up, that man also has missed the
way. These are the two extremes, the two mistakes
at the two ends. Both have lost the way, both have
missed the goal.

So work, says Vedānta, putting God in everything
and knowing Him to be in everything. Work incessantly, holding life as something deified, as God Himself, and knowing that this is all we have to do, this
is all we should ask for. God is in everything; where
else shall we go to find Him? He is already in every
work, in every thought, in every feeling. Knowing
this, we must work. This is the only way; there is no
other. The effects of work will then not bind us. We
have seen that false desires are the cause of all the
misery and evil we suffer from; but when they are
thus deified, purified, through God, they bring no
evil, they bring no misery. Those who have not learnt

this secret will have to live in a demoniacal world until they discover it. Many do not know what an infinite mine of bliss is in them, around them, everywhere; they have not yet discovered it. What is a demoniacal world? Ignorance, says Vedānta.

We are dying of thirst sitting on the bank of the mightiest river. We are dying of hunger sitting near heaps of food. Here is the blissful universe; yet we do not find it. We are in it all the time and we are always misjudging it. Religion proposes to find this out for us. The longing for this blissful universe is in all hearts. It has been the search of all nations, it is the one goal of religion, and this ideal is expressed in various languages in different religions. It is only the difference of language that makes all these apparent divergences: one expresses a thought in one way, another a little differently, yet perhaps each means exactly what the other is expressing in a different language.

More questions arise in connexion with this. It is very easy to talk. From my childhood I have been told that I should see God everywhere and in everything, and then I could really enjoy the world; but as soon as I mix with the world and get a few blows from it, the idea vanishes. I am walking in the street thinking that God is in every man, and a strong man comes along and gives me a push and I fall flat on the footpath. Then I rise up quickly with clenched fist, the blood has rushed to my head, and my discrimination goes. Immediately I have become mad. Everything is forgotten; instead of encountering God I see the Devil. Ever since we were born we have been told to see God

in all. Every religion teaches that: see God in everything and everywhere. Do you not remember that
in the New Testament Christ says so? We have all
been taught that; but it is when we come to the
practical side that the difficulty begins.

You remember reading in *Aesop's Fables* about a
fine stag looking at his form reflected in a lake and
saying to his young one: "How powerful I am! Look
at my splendid head; look at my limbs. How strong
and muscular they are! And how swiftly I can run!"
Then he hears the barking of dogs in the distance
and immediately takes to his heels; and after he has
run several miles he comes back panting. The young
one says: "You just told me how strong you were.
How was it that when the dogs barked you ran away?"
"Yes, my son; but when the dogs bark all my con-
fidence vanishes." Such is the case with us. We think
highly of humanity, we feel ourselves strong and
valiant, we make grand resolves; but when the dogs of
trials and temptations bark, we are like the stag in
the fable.

Then, if such is the case, what is the use of teaching all these things? There is the greatest use. The
use is this: that perseverance will finally conquer.
Nothing can be done in a day.

"This Self is first to be heard about, then to be
thought upon, and then meditated upon." Everyone
can see the sky; even the very worm crawling upon
the earth sees the blue sky—but how very far away
it is! So it is with our ideal. It is far away, no doubt,
but at the same time we know that we must have it.
We must have the highest ideal. Unfortunately, in

this world the vast majority of persons are groping in the dark without any ideal at all. If a man with an ideal makes a thousand mistakes, I am sure that the man without an ideal makes fifty thousand. Therefore it is better to have an ideal. And this ideal we must hear about as much as we can, till it enters into our hearts, into our brains, into our very veins, till it tingles in every drop of our blood and permeates every pore in our body. We must meditate upon it. "Out of the fullness of the heart the mouth speaketh," and out of the fullness of the heart the hand works, too.

It is thought which is the propelling force in us. Fill the mind with the highest thoughts, hear them day after day, think them month after month. Never mind failures; they are quite natural. They are the beauty of life, these failures. What would life be without them? It would not be worth having if it were not for struggles. Where would be the poetry of life? Never mind the struggles, the mistakes. I never heard a cow tell a lie; but it is only a cow— not a man. So never mind these failures, these little backslidings; hold to the ideal a thousand times, and if you fail a thousand times, make the attempt once more. The ideal of man is to see God in everything. But if you cannot see Him in everything, see Him in one thing, in that thing which you like best, and then see Him in another. So on you can go. There is infinite life before the soul. Take your time and you will achieve your end.

"He, the One, who vibrates more quickly than the mind, who attains more speed than the mind can ever attain, whom even the gods reach not, nor thought grasps—He moving, everything moves. In Him all exists. He is moving; He is also immovable. He is near and He is far. He is inside everything, He is outside everything—interpenetrating everything. Whoever sees in every being that same Ātman, and whoever sees everything in that Ātman, he never goes far from that Ātman. When a man sees all life and the whole universe in this Ātman, then he does not become secretive. There is no more delusion for him. Where is any more misery for him who sees this Oneness in the universe?"

This is another great theme of Vedānta, this Oneness of life, this Oneness of everything. We shall see how it demonstrates that all our misery comes through ignorance, and that this ignorance is nothing but the idea of manifoldness, of separation between man and man, between nation and nation, between earth and moon, between moon and sun. Out of this idea of separation between atom and atom comes all misery. But Vedānta says that this separation does not exist; it is not real. It is merely apparent, on the surface. In the heart of things there is unity. If you go below the surface you find that unity between man and man, between race and race, high and low, rich and poor, gods and men, men and animals. If you go deep enough all will be seen as only variations of the One.

He who has attained to this conception of Oneness has no more delusion. What can delude him? He knows the reality of everything, the secret of everything. Where is there any more misery for him? What

does he desire? He has traced the reality of everything to the Lord, who is the Centre of all things,
and who is Eternal Existence, Eternal Knowledge,
Eternal Bliss. Neither death nor disease nor sorrow
nor misery nor discontent is there. All is Perfect
Union and Perfect Bliss. For whom should he mourn
then? In reality there is no death, there is no misery;
in reality there is no one to mourn for, no one to
be sorry for. He has penetrated everything—He, the
Pure One, the Formless, the Bodiless, the Stainless—
He, the Knower—He, the Great Poet, the Self-
existent—He who gives to everyone what he deserves.

They grope in darkness who worship this material
world, the world that is produced out of ignorance,
thinking of it as Brahman, and those who live their
whole lives in this world and never find anything
better or higher are groping in still greater darkness.
But he who knows the secret of nature, and also That
which is beyond nature—through the help of nature
he crosses death, and through the help of That which
is beyond nature he enjoys Eternal Bliss.

"The door of the Truth is covered by a golden
disc. Open it, O Nourisher! Remove it so that I who
have been worshipping the Truth may behold It.

"O Nourisher, lone Traveller of the sky! Controller!
O Sun, Offspring of Prajāpati! Gather Your rays;
withdraw Your light. I would see, through Your
grace, that form of Yours which is the fairest. I am
indeed He, that Purusha, who dwells there."

UNITY IN DIVERSITY

(Delivered in London, November 3, 1896)

"THE SELF-EXISTENT ONE projected the senses outward and therefore a man looks outward, not within himself. A certain wise one, desiring immortality, turned the senses inward and perceived the Self within." As I have already said, the first inquiry in the Vedas was concerning outward things; and then a new idea came: that the reality of things is not to be found in the external world; it is to be found not by looking outward, but by turning the eyes, as it is expressed literally, inward. And the word used for the Soul is very significant: it is He who has gone inward, the innermost reality of our being, the heart centre, the core from which, as it were, everything comes out; the central Sun, of which the mind, the body, the sense-organs, and everything else that we have are but rays going outward.

"Men of childish intellect, ignorant persons, run after desires, which are external, and enter the trap of far-reaching death; but the wise, understanding immortality, never seek the Eternal in this life of finite things." The same idea is here made clear, that in this external world, which is full of finite things, it is impossible to see and find the Infinite. The Infinite must be sought in that alone which is infinite, and the only thing infinite about us is that which is within us, our own Soul. Neither the body nor the mind, not

88

even our thoughts nor the world we see around us, is infinite. The Seer, He to whom they all belong, the Soul of man, He who is awake in the internal man, alone is infinite; and to seek the infinite Cause of this whole universe we must go *there*. In the infinite Soul alone can we find It.

"What is here is there too, and what is there is also here. He who sees the manifold goes from death to death."

We have seen how at first there was the desire to go to heaven. When the ancient Āryans became dissatisfied with the world around them, they naturally thought that after death they would go to certain places where there would be all happiness without any misery; these places they called svargas—the word may be translated as heavens—where there would be joy for ever; the body would become perfect, and also the mind, and there they would live with their forefathers.

But as soon as philosophy came men found that this was impossible and absurd. The very idea of something infinite in any place would be a contradiction in terms, as a place must begin and continue in time. Therefore they had to give up that idea. They found out that the gods who lived in these heavens were human beings who through their good works on earth had become gods, and that these various divinities were different states, different positions.

None of the gods spoken of in the Vedas are permanent individuals. For instance, Indra and Varuna are not the names of certain persons, but the names of positions as governors and so on. The Indra who lived before is not the same person as the Indra of the present day; he has passed away, and another man from earth has filled his place. So with all the other gods. These are certain positions, which are filled successively by human souls who have raised themselves to the condition of gods; and yet even they die.

In the old Rig-Veda we find the word *immortality* used with regard to these gods; but later it was dropped entirely, for it was found that true immortality, which is beyond time and space, cannot be spoken of with regard to any physical form, however subtle, however fine it may be. It must have had a beginning in time and space; for the necessary factors that enter into the make-up of form are in space. Try to think of having form without space. It is impossible. Space is one of the materials, as it were, which make up the form, and this form is continually changing. Space and time are in māyā, and this idea is expressed in the line: "What is here is there too." If there are these gods they must be bound by the same laws that apply here, and all these laws involve destruction and re-newal again and again. These laws are moulding mat-ter into different forms and crushing them out again. Everything born must die; and so if there are heavens, the same laws must hold good there.

In this world we find that all happiness is followed by misery as its shadow. Life has its shadow, death. They must go together, because they are not contra-dictory, not two separate existences, but different mani-festations of the same unit, which appears as both life and death, sorrow and happiness, good and evil. The dualistic conception that good and evil are two separate entities, and that they both continue eternally, is absurd on the face of it. They are the diverse manifestations of one and the same fact, one time appearing as bad and another time as good. The difference is not one of kind but only of degree. They differ from each other in intensity.

We find, as a matter of fact, that the same nerve systems carry good and bad sensations alike, and when the nerves are injured neither sensation comes to us. If a certain nerve is paralysed we do not get the pleasurable feelings that used to come along that wire, and at the same time we do not get the painful feelings either. They are not essentially different. Again, the same thing produces pleasure and pain at different times of life. The same phenomenon will produce pleasure in one and pain in another. The eating of meat produces pleasure in a man, but pain in the animal which is eaten. There has never been anything which gives pleasure to all alike. Some are pleased, others displeased. So it will go on.

Therefore this duality of existence is denied. And what follows? I told you in my last lecture that we can never ultimately have everything good on this earth and nothing bad. It may have disappointed and frightened some of you, but I cannot help it and I am open to conviction if I am shown the contrary; but until that can be proved to me, I cannot accept it.

The general argument against my statement, and apparently a very convincing one, is that in the course of evolution all that is evil in what we see around us is gradually being eliminated, and that if this process of elimination continues for millions of years, a time will come when all the evil will have been extirpated and the good alone will remain. This is apparently a very sound argument. Would to God it were true! But there is a fallacy in it and it is this: It takes for granted that both good and evil are entities that are eternally fixed. It takes for granted that there is a definite mass of evil which may be represented by a hundred, and likewise a definite mass of good, and that this mass of evil is being diminished every day, leaving only the good. But is it so? The history of the world shows that evil, as well as good, is a continuously increasing quantity. Take the lowest man. He lives in the forest. His power of enjoyment is very small, and so also is his power to suffer. His misery is entirely on the sense plane. If he does not get plenty of food he is miserable; but give him plenty of food and freedom to rove and to hunt, and he is perfectly happy. His happiness is only in the senses, and so is his misery. But if that man's knowledge increases, his happiness too will increase, his intellect will develop, and his sense enjoyment will evolve into intellectual enjoyment. He will feel pleasure in reading a beautiful poem, and a mathematical problem will be of absorbing interest to him. But along with this the finer nerves will become more and more susceptible to the miseries of mental pain, about which the savage does not think.

Take another very simple illustration. In certain parts of Tibet there is no marriage as we understand it, and therefore no jealousy; yet we know that marriage is a much higher state. These Tibetans have not known the wonderful joy of chastity, the happiness of being blessed with a chaste, virtuous wife or a chaste, virtuous husband. These people cannot feel that. And similarly they do not feel the intense jealousy of the chaste wife or husband, or the misery caused by unfaithfulness on either side, with all the heart-burnings and sorrows which believers in chastity experience. On one side they gain in happiness, but on the other they suffer misery too.

Take your country, which is the richest in the world, and which is more luxurious than any other, and see how intense is the misery, how much more insanity you have, compared with other races, only because the desires are so keen. A man must keep up a high standard of living, and the amount of money he spends in one year would be a fortune to a man in India. You cannot preach to an Englishman about simple living, because society demands so much of him. The wheel of society is rolling on; it stops not for the widows' tears or the orphans' wails. This is the state of things everywhere. Your power of enjoyment is developed; your society is very much more beautiful than some others. You have so many more things to enjoy. But those who have fewer have much less misery.

You can argue thus throughout. The higher the ideal you have, the greater is your enjoyment and also the more profound your misery. One is like the shadow of the other. That the evils are being eliminated may be true, but if so, the good also must be dying out. But are not the evils multiplying fast, and the good diminishing, if I may so put it? If good increases in arithmetical proportion, evil increases in geometrical proportion. And this is māyā.

This is neither optimism nor pessimism. Vedānta does not take the position that this world is only a miserable one. That would be untrue. On the other hand, it would also be a mistake to say that this world is full of happiness and blessings. So it is useless to tell children that this world is all good, all flowers and milk and honey—which is what we have all dreamt. At the same time it is erroneous to think that because one man has suffered more than another, all is evil. It is this duality, this play of good and evil, that makes our world of experience. Nevertheless, Vedānta says, we should not think that good and evil are two separate entities; for they are one and the same thing appearing in different degrees and in different guises and producing differences of feeling in the same mind. So the first thought of Vedānta is the finding of unity in the external—the One Existence manifesting Itself, however differently It may appear in Its manifestations.

Think of the old theory of the Persians: two gods creating this world, the good god doing everything that is good, and the bad one everything that is bad. On the very face of it, you see the absurdity; for if it is carried out, every law of nature must have two parts, one of which is manipulated by one god, who then goes away while the other god manipulates the other part. There the difficulty comes: both are working in the same world, and these two gods keep in harmony by injuring one portion and doing good to another. This is a crude case, of course, the crudest way of expressing the duality of existence. But take the more advanced, the more abstract theory, that this world is partly good and partly bad. This also is absurd, arguing from the same standpoint. It is the same force that provides us with our food and that kills many through accidents or misadventures.

We find, then, that this world is neither good nor evil; it is a mixture of both. And as we go on we shall see that Vedānta takes the whole blame away from nature and puts it upon our own shoulders. At the same time Vedānta shows the way out—but not by the denial of evil, because it boldly analyses the fact as it is and does not seek to conceal anything. It is not a creed of hopelessness; it is not agnosticism. It has found out a solution of the problem of good and evil, and has placed that solution on such adamantine foundations that it does not gag men, as if they were mere children, and blind their eyes with something which is untrue and which they will find out about in a few days.

I remember when I was young, a young man's father died and left him poorly off, with a large family to support, and he found that his father's friends were unwilling to help him. He had a conversation with a clergyman, who offered this consolation, "Oh, it is all good; all is done for our good." That is the old method of trying to put a piece of gold-leaf on an old sore. It is a confession of weakness, of ignorance. The young man went away, and six months afterwards a son was born to the clergyman, and he gave a thanksgiving party to which the young man was invited. The clergyman prayed, "Thank God for His mercies." And the young man stood up and said, "Stop! This is all misery." The clergyman asked, "Why?" "Because when my father died you said it was good, though apparently evil; so now this is apparently good, but really evil."

Is that the way to cure the misery of the world? Do not
try to patch it up; nothing will cure this world. Go
beyond it.

This is a world of good and evil. Wherever there
is good, evil follows; but beyond and behind all these
manifestations, all these contradictions, Vedānta finds
Unity; and it says, "Give up what is evil and give up
what is good." What then remains? Behind good and
evil stands something which is yours, the real "you"
—beyond every evil, and beyond every good too—and
it is that which is manifesting itself as good and evil.

Know that first; then, and then alone, will you be a
true optimist, and not before; for then you will be
able to control everything. Control these manifestations
and you will be at liberty to manifest the real "you."
First be master of yourself, stand up and be free, go
beyond the pale of these laws; for these laws do not
absolutely govern you; they are only part of your being.
First find out that you are not the slave of nature,
never were and never will be; that this nature, infinite
as you may think it, is only finite, a drop in the ocean,
and your Soul is the ocean. You are beyond the stars,
the sun, and the moon. They are like mere bubbles
compared with your infinite Being. Know that, and
you will control both good and evil. Then alone will
your whole vision change, and you will stand up and
say, "How beautiful is good and how wonderful is
evil!"

That is what Vedānta teaches. It does not propose
any slipshod remedy by covering wounds with gold-
leaf, and the more the wound festers, putting on more
gold-leaf. This life is a hard fact. Work your way

through it boldly, though it may be adamantine. No matter! The soul is stronger. Vedānta lays no responsibility on little gods; for you are the makers of your own fortunes. You make yourselves suffer, you make good and evil, and it is you who put your hands before your eyes and say it is dark. Take your hands away and see the light; you are effulgent, you are perfect already, from the very beginning.

We now understand the verse: "He goes from death to death who sees the many here." See that Oneness and be free. How are we to see it? This mind, so deluded, so weak, so easily led, even this mind can be strong and can catch a glimpse of that Knowledge, that Oneness, which saves us from dying again and again.

As rain falling upon a mountain flows in various streams down the sides of the mountain, so all the energies which you see here are from that one Centre. It has become manifold falling upon māyā. Do not run after the manifold; go towards the One. "He is in all that moves; He is in all that is pure. He fills the universe. He is in the sacrifice; He is the guest in the house; He is in man, in water, in animals, in truth; He is the Great One. As fire coming into this world manifests itself in various forms, even so that one Soul of the universe manifests Himself in all these various forms. As air coming into this universe manifests itself in various forms, even so the one Soul of all souls, of all beings, manifests Himself in all forms." This is true for you when you have understood this Unity, and not before. Then all is optimism, because He is seen everywhere.

The question is: If this be true—that that Pure

One, the Self, the Infinite, has entered all this—how is it that He suffers, how is it that He becomes miserable, impure? He does not, says the Upanishad. "As the sun is the cause of the eyesight of every being, yet is not made defective by the defect in any eye, even so the Self of all is not affected by the miseries of the body, or by any misery in the world." I may have some disease and see everything yellow, but the sun is not affected by it.

"He is the One, the Creator of all, the Ruler of all, the Internal Soul of every being, He who makes His Oneness manifold. Thus sages who realize Him as the Soul of their souls—unto them belongs eternal peace; unto none else, unto none else. He who in this world of evanescence finds Him who never changes, he who in this universe of death finds that One Life, he who in this manifold finds that Oneness, he who realizes Him as the Soul of his soul—unto him belongs eternal peace; unto none else, unto none else." How can one find Him in the external world? How can one find Him in the sun or moon or stars? "There the sun cannot shine, nor the moon, nor the stars; the flash of lightning cannot illumine Him, not to speak of this mortal fire. He shining, everything else shines. It is His light that they have borrowed, and He is shining through them."

Here is another beautiful passage from the *Katha Upanishad*: "This is that eternal Aśvattha Tree with its root above and branches below. That root, indeed, is called the Bright; That is Brahman, and That alone is the Immortal. In That all worlds are contained, and none can pass beyond."

Various heavens are spoken of in the Brāhmana portion of the Vedas, but the philosophical teaching of the Upanishads discourages the idea of going to heaven. Happiness is not in this heaven or in that heaven; it is in the soul. Places do not signify anything.

Here is another passage, which shows the different states of realization: "In the heaven of the forefathers, as a man sees things in a dream, so the Real Truth is seen." As in dreams we see things hazy and not distinct, so we see Reality there. There is another heaven, called the Gandharvaloka, in which Reality is seen as a man sees his own reflection in water. The highest heaven of which the Hindus conceive is called Brahmaloka; and there Truth is seen much more clearly, like light and shade, but not yet quite distinctly. But as a man sees his own face in a mirror, perfect, distinct, and clear, so does Truth shine in the soul of man.

The highest heaven, therefore, is in our own souls; the greatest temple of worship is the human soul, greater than all heavens, says Vedānta; for in no heaven, anywhere, can we understand Reality as distinctly and clearly as in this life, in our own soul.

Changing places does not help one much. I thought while I was in India that a cave would give me clearer vision. I found it was not so. Then I thought the forest would do so. Then, Benares. But the same difficulty existed everywhere, because we make our own world. If I am evil, the whole world is evil to me; that is what the Upanishad says. And the same thing applies to all worlds. If I die and go to heaven, I shall find the

same; for until I am pure it is no use going to caves
or forests or to Benares or to heaven; and if I have
polished my mirror, it does not matter where I live;
I see Reality just as It is. So it is useless running hither
and thither and spending energy in vain, which should
be spent only in polishing the mirror. The same idea
is expressed again: "None sees Him, none sees His
form with the eyes. It is in the mind, in the pure mind,
that He is seen, and thus immortality is gained."

Those who were at the summer lectures on rāja-yoga
will be interested to know that what was taught then
was a different kind of yoga. The yoga which we are
now considering consists chiefly in controlling the
senses. When the senses are held as slaves by the
human soul, when they can no longer disturb the
mind, then the yogi has reached the goal. "When all
vain desires of the heart have been given up, then this
very mortal becomes immortal, then he becomes one
with God even here. When all the knots of the heart
are cut asunder, then the mortal becomes immortal
and he enjoys Brahman here." Here on this earth—
nowhere else.

A few words ought to be said here. You will generally hear that this Vedānta philosophy and other
Eastern systems look only to something beyond, letting
go the enjoyments and struggles of this life. This idea
is entirely wrong. It is only ignorant people who do
not know anything of Eastern thought and never had
brain enough to understand anything of its real teaching, who tell you so. On the contrary, we read in our
scriptures that our philosophers do not want us to go
to other worlds, but depreciate them as places where

people laugh for a little while only and then die. As long as we are weak we shall have to go through these experiences of heaven and hell; but whatever is true is here, and that is the human soul. And this also is insisted upon: by committing suicide we cannot escape the inevitable chain of birth and death. But the right path is hard to find.

The Hindu is just as practical as the Westerner, only they differ in their views of life. The one says, "Build a good house, have good clothes and food, intellectual culture, and so on, for this is the whole of life"; and in that he is immensely practical. But the Hindu says, "True knowledge of the world means knowledge of the soul, metaphysics"; and he wants to enjoy that life.

In America there was a great agnostic, a very noble man, a very good man, and a very fine speaker. He lectured on religion, which he said was of no use; why bother our heads about other worlds? He employed this metaphor: "We have an orange here, and we want to squeeze all the juice out of it." I met him once and said: "I agree with you entirely. I have some fruit and I too want to squeeze out the juice. Our difference lies in the choice of the fruit. You want an orange, and I prefer a mango. You think it is enough to live here and eat and drink and have a little scientific knowledge, but you have no right to say that that will suit all tastes. Such a conception is nothing to me. If I had only to learn how an apple falls to the ground or how an electric current shakes my nerves, I should commit suicide. I want to understand the heart of things, the very kernel itself. Your study is the manifestation of life; mine is life itself. My philosophy says you must know *that* and drive out from your mind all thoughts of heaven and hell and all other superstitions, even though they exist in the same sense that this world exists. I must know the heart of this life, its very essence, what it is—not merely how it works and what are its manifestations. I want the *why* of everything; I leave the *how* to children. It was one of your countrymen who said, 'If I were to write a book about what I feel when I smoke a cigarette, it would be the science of the cigarette.' It is good and great to be scientific. God bless the scientists in their search! But if one says that that is all, one is talking foolishly, not caring to know the meaning of life, never studying existence itself. I can prove that all your knowledge is nonsense, without a basis. You are studying the manifestation of life, and when I ask you what life is, you say you do not know. You are welcome to your study, but leave me to mine."

I am practical, very practical, in my own way. So your idea that only the West is practical is nonsense. You are practical in one way, and I in another. There are different types of men and minds. If in the East a man is told that he will find out the truth by standing on one leg all his life, he will pursue that method. If in the West men hear that there is a gold-mine somewhere in an uncivilized country, thousands will face the dangers there in the hope of getting the gold; and perhaps only one succeeds. The same men have heard that they have souls, but are content to leave the care of them to the church. The Easterner will not go near the savages; he says it may be dangerous. But if we tell him that on the top of a high mountain lives a wonderful sage who can give him knowledge of the soul, he tries to climb up to him, even though he may be killed in the attempt. Both types of men are practical; but the mistake lies in regarding this world as the whole of life. Yours is the evanescent enjoyment of the senses; there is nothing permanent in it; it only brings more and more misery. But mine is eternal peace.

I do not say your view is wrong. You are welcome to it. Great good and blessing come out of it. But do not on that account condemn my view. Mine also is practical in its own way. Let us all work on our own plan. Would to God all of us were equally practical on both sides! I have seen some scientists who are equally practical as scientists and as spiritual men, and it is my great hope that in the course of time the whole of humanity will be efficient in the same manner.

When a kettle of water is coming to the boil, if you watch the phenomenon you find first one bubble rising and then another, and so on, until at last they all join and a tremendous commotion takes place. This world is very similar. Each individual is like a bubble, and the nations resemble many bubbles. Gradually these nations are joining, and I am sure the day will come when separation will vanish and that Oneness to which we are all going will become manifest. A time must come when every man will be as intensely practical in the spiritual world as in the scientific, and then that Oneness, the harmony of Oneness, will pervade the whole world. The whole of mankind will become jivanmuktas—free while living. We are all struggling towards that one end through our jealousies and

hatreds, through our love and co-operation. A tremendous stream is flowing towards the ocean, carrying
us all along with it; and though, like straws and
scraps of paper, we may at times float aimlessly about,
in the long run we are sure to join the Ocean of Life
and Bliss.

THE FREEDOM OF THE SOUL

(Delivered in London, November 5, 1896)

THE *Katha Upanishad,* which we have been studying, was written much later than that to which
we now turn—the *Chhāndogya;* the language of the
former is more modern and the thought more organized. In the older Upanishads the language is very
archaic, like that of the hymn portion of the Vedas,
and one has to wade sometimes through quite a mass
of unnecessary things to get at the essential doctrines.
The ritualistic literature of the Vedas, about which I
have told you, has greatly influenced this old Upanishad, so that more than half of it is still ritualistic.
There is, however, one great gain in studying the very
old Upanishads. You trace, as it were, the historical
growth of spiritual ideas. In the more recent Upanishads the spiritual ideas have been collected and
brought into one place; in the Bhagavad Gitā, for
instance, which we may perhaps look upon as the last
of the Upanishads, you do not find any inkling of these
ritualistic ideas. The Gitā is like a bouquet composed
of the beautiful flowers of spiritual truths collected
from the Upanishads. But in the Gitā you cannot
study the growth of the spiritual ideas; you cannot
trace them to their source. To do that, as has been
pointed out by many, you must study the Vedas.

The idea of great holiness that has been attached
to these books has preserved them, more than any other

book in the world, from mutilation. In them, thoughts
at their highest and at their lowest have all been preserved—the essential and the non-essential. The most
ennobling teachings and the simplest matters of detail
stand side by side; for nobody has dared to touch them.
Commentators came and tried to smooth them down
and bring out wonderful new ideas from the old things;
they tried to find spiritual ideas in even the most
ordinary statements; but the texts remained, and these
texts are the most wonderful historical study. We all
know that in the scriptures of every religion changes
were made to suit the growing spirituality of later
times; one word was changed here and another put
in there, and so on. This probably has not been done
with the Vedic literature, or if ever done, it is almost
imperceptible. So we have this great advantage: we
are able to study thoughts in their original significance,
to note how they developed, how from materialistic
ideas finer and finer spiritual ideas evolved, until they
attained their greatest height in Vedānta. Descriptions
of some of the old manners and customs are also to be
found in the Vedic literature; but they do not appear
much in the Upanishads, where the language used is
a peculiarly terse mnemonic.

The writers of these books simply jotted down these
lines as helps to remember certain facts which they
supposed were already well known. In a narrative
which they are telling, they perhaps take it for granted
that it is well known to everyone they are addressing.
Thus a great difficulty arises: we scarcely know the
real meaning of any one of these stories, because the
traditions have nearly died out, and the little that is

left of them has been very much exaggerated. Many new interpretations have been put upon them, so that when you find them in the Purānas they have already become lyrical poems.

Just as in the West we find, in the political development of the Western races, the prominent fact that they cannot bear absolute rule, that they are always trying to prevent any one man from ruling over them and are gradually advancing to higher and higher democratic ideas, higher and higher ideas of physical liberty, so, in Indian metaphysics, exactly the same phenomenon appears in the development of the spiritual life. The multiplicity of gods gave place to one God of the universe, and in the Upanishads there is a rebellion even against that one God. The idea was unbearable not only that there should be many governors of the universe ruling their destinies, but also that there should be one person ruling this universe. This is the first thing that strikes us. The idea grows and grows, until it attains its climax. In almost all the Upanishads we find the climax coming at the last, and that is the dethroning of this God of the universe. The personality of God vanishes; impersonality comes. God is no more a person, no more a human being, however magnified and exaggerated, who rules this universe, but He has become an embodied principle in every being, immanent in the whole universe.

It would be illogical to go from the Personal God to the Impersonal and at the same time leave man as a person. So the personal man is broken down, and man as a principle is built up. The person is only a phenomenon; the principle is behind it. Thus from both

sides, simultaneously, we find the breaking down of
personalities and the approach towards principles, the
Personal God approaching the Impersonal, the personal
man approaching the impersonal man. Then come the
succeeding stages—the gradual convergence of the two
advancing lines of the Impersonal God and the impersonal man. And the Upanishads embody the stages
through which these two lines at last become one; and
the last word of each Upanishad is "Thou art That."
There is but one eternally blissful Principle, and that
One is manifesting Itself as all this variety.

Then came the philosophers. The work of the
Upanishads seems to have ended at that point; the
next step was taken by the philosophers. The frame-
work was given them by the Upanishads, and they had
to fill in the details. Many questions would naturally
arise. Taking for granted that there is but one Impersonal Principle, which is manifesting Itself in all these
manifold forms, how is it that the One becomes many?
It is another way of putting the same old question
which in its crude form comes into the human heart
as the inquiry into the cause of evil and so forth. Why
does evil exist in the world, and what is its cause? But
the same question has now become refined, abstracted.
No more is it asked from the sense plane why we are
unhappy; but it is asked from the plane of philosophy:
Why has this one Principle become manifold? And the
answer, as we have seen, the best answer that India
has produced, is the theory of māyā, which says that
It really has not become manifold, that It really has
not lost any of Its real nature. Manifoldness is only
apparent. Man is only apparently a person, but in

reality he is Impersonal Being. God is a Person only apparently, but really He is Impersonal Being.

But even in the finding out of this answer there have been succeeding stages, and philosophers have varied in their opinions. Not all Indian philosophers have accepted this theory of māyā. Possibly most of them have not. There are dualists, with a crude sort of dualism, who will not allow the question to be asked, but stifle it at the very outset. They say: "You have no right to ask such a question; you have no right to ask for an explanation. It is simply the will of God, and we have to submit to it quietly. There is no liberty for the human soul. Everything is predes-tined—what we shall do, have, enjoy, and suffer; and when suffering comes it is our duty to endure it patiently. If we do not, we shall be punished all the more. How do we know that? Because the Vedas say so." And thus they quote their texts and give their meanings and they want to enforce them.

There are others who, though not admitting the māyā theory, stand midway. They say that the whole of this creation forms, as it were, the body of God. God is the Soul of all souls and of the whole of nature. In the case of individual souls, contraction comes from evil-doing. When a man does anything evil his soul begins to contract and his power is diminished and goes on decreasing, until he does good works, when it expands again.

One idea seems to be common to all the Indian sys-tems, and I think to all the systems in the world, whether they know it or not, and that is what I should call the divinity of man. There is not one system in

the world, not one religion, which does not hold the
idea—whether expressed in the language of mythology,
allegory, or philosophy—that the human soul, whatever it be, or whatever its relation to God, is essentially
pure and perfect. Its real nature is blessedness and
power, not weakness and misery. Somehow this present misery has come. The crude systems may speak of
a personified evil, a Devil, or an Ahriman, to explain
how this misery came. Other systems may try to make
a God and a Devil in one, who makes some people
miserable and others happy, without any reason whatever. Others again, more thoughtful, bring in the
theory of māyā, and so forth. But one thing stands
out clearly, and it is with this that we have to deal.
After all, these philosophical ideas and systems are but
gymnastics of the mind, intellectual exercises. The one
great idea that to me seems to be clear and that comes
out through masses of superstition in every country
and in every religion is the luminous idea that man is
divine, that divinity is our nature.

Whatever else comes is a mere superimposition, as
Vedānta calls it. Something has been superimposed,
but that cannot kill the divine nature. In the most degraded, as well as in the most saintly, it is ever present.
It has to be called out and it will work itself out. We
have to ask and it will manifest itself. The people of
old knew that fire existed in flint and in dry wood,
but friction was necessary to call it out. So this fire of
freedom and purity is the nature of every soul, and is
not a quality, because qualities can be acquired and
therefore can be lost.

The soul is one with Freedom, and the soul is one

with Existence, and the soul is one with Knowledge. Satchidānanda, Existence-Knowledge-Bliss Absolute, is the nature, the birthright, of the soul, and all the manifestations that we see are Its expressions, dimly or brightly manifesting It. Even death is but a manifestation of that Real Existence. Birth and death, life and decay, degeneration and regeneration, are all manifestations of that Oneness. So knowledge, however it manifests itself, either as ignorance or as learning, is but the manifestation of that same Chit, the Essence of Knowledge; the difference is only in degree and not in kind. The difference in knowledge between the lowest worm that crawls under our feet and the highest genius that the world may produce is only one of degree and not of kind. The Vedāntist thinker boldly says that the enjoyments in this life, even the most degraded joys, are but manifestations of that one Divine Bliss, the Essence of the soul.

This idea seems to be the most prominent in Vedānta, and, as I have said, it appears to me that every religion holds it. I have yet to know the religion which does not. It is the one universal idea working through all religions.

Take the Bible, for instance. You find there the allegorical statement that the first man, Adam, was pure, and that afterwards his purity was obliterated by his evil deeds. It is clear from this allegory that the Hebrews thought that the original nature of man was perfect; the impurities that we see, the weaknesses that we feel, are but superimpositions on that nature. And the subsequent history of the Christian religion shows that the Christians believe in the possibility, nay, the certainty, of regaining that old state. This is the whole history of the Bible, Old and New Testaments together.

So it is with the Mohammedans. They also believe in Adam and the purity of Adam, and hold that through Mohammed the way has been opened to regain that lost state.

So, too, with the Buddhists. They believe in the state called Nirvāna, which is beyond this relative world. It is exactly the same as the Brahman of the Vedāntists; and the whole system of Buddhism is founded upon the idea of regaining that lost state of Nirvāna.

In every system we find this doctrine present—that you cannot get anything which is not yours already. You are indebted to nobody in this universe. You claim your own birthright—as it has been poetically expressed by a great Vedāntist in the title of one of his books, *Swārājyasiddhi, The Attainment of Our Own Empire.* That empire is ours; we have lost it and we have to regain it. The māyāvādin, however, says that the idea of having lost the empire is a hallucination; you never lost it. This is the only difference.

Although all the systems agree so far—that we had the empire and that we have lost it—they give us varied advice as to how to regain it. One says that we must perform certain ceremonies, worship certain deities in a certain way, eat certain sorts of food, live in a peculiar fashion, to regain that empire. Another says that if we weep and prostrate ourselves and ask pardon of some Being beyond nature, we shall regain that empire. Again, another says that if we love such a Being with all our heart, we shall regain that empire. All this varied advice is in the Upanishads. As I go on, you will find it so.

But the last and the greatest counsel is that we need not weep at all. We need not go through all these ceremonies and need not take any notice of how to regain our empire, because we never lost it. Why should we go about seeking what we never lost? We are pure already, we are free already. If we think we are free, free we are this moment, and if we think we are bound, bound we shall be.

This is a very bold statement, and as I told you at the beginning of these lectures, I shall have to speak to you very boldly. It may frighten you now; but when you think it over and realize it in your own life, then you will come to know that what I say is true. If that freedom is not your nature, by no manner of means can you become free. Or if you were free and in some way you lost that freedom, then you were not free to begin with. Had you been free, what could have made you lose it? The independent can never be made dependent; if it is really dependent, its independence was a hallucination.

Of the two sides, then, which will you take? If you say that the soul was by its own nature pure and free, it naturally follows that there was nothing in this universe which could make it bound or limited. But if there was anything in nature which could bind the soul, it naturally follows that it was not free, and your statement that it was free is a delusion. So if it is possible for us to attain to freedom, the conclusion is inevitable that the soul is by its nature free. It cannot be otherwise.

Freedom means independence of anything outside, and that means that nothing outside itself could work upon it as a cause. The soul is causeless, and from this follow all the great ideas that we have. You cannot establish the immortality of the soul unless you grant that it is by its nature free, or in other words, that it cannot be acted upon by anything outside; for death is an effect produced by some outside cause. I drink poison and I die, thus showing that my body can be acted upon by something outside that is called poison. But if it be true that the soul is free, it naturally follows that nothing can affect it and it can never die. The freedom, immortality, and blessedness of the soul have meaning only if it is beyond the law of causation.

Of these two, which will you take? Either make the first a delusion or make the second a delusion. Certainly I will make the second a delusion. It is more consonant with all my feelings and aspirations. I am perfectly aware that I am free by nature, and I will not admit that this bondage is true and my freedom a delusion.

This discussion goes on, in some form or other, in all philosophies. Even in the most modern philosophies you find the same discussion. There are two parties. One says that there is no soul, that the idea of the soul is a delusion produced by the rapid succession of particles of matter, bringing about the combination which you call the body or the brain; that the impression of freedom is the result of the vibrations and motions and continuous succession of these particles. There were Buddhist sects who held the same view and illustrated it by this example: If you take a torch and whirl it round rapidly, there will be a circle of light. That circle does not really exist, because the torch is changing place every moment. We are but bundles of little particles, which in their rapid whirling produce the delusion of a permanent soul.

The other party states that the rapid succession of thought creates the delusion of matter, which does not really exist. So we see one side claiming that spirit is a delusion, and the other that matter is a delusion. Which side will you take? Of course we will take spirit and deny matter. The arguments are similar for both; only on the spirit side the argument is a little stronger. For nobody has ever seen what matter is; we can only feel ourselves. I never knew a man who could feel matter by going outside of himself. Nobody was ever able to jump outside of himself. Therefore the argument is a little stronger on the side of the spirit. Secondly, the spirit theory explains the universe, while materialism does not. Hence the materialistic explanation is illogical. If you boil down all the philosophies and analyse them, you will find that they are reduced to one or other of these two positions.

So here, too, in a more intricate form, in a more philosophical form, we find the same question about freedom and bondage. One side says that the first is a delusion, and the other that the second is a delusion. And of course we side with the second in believing that our bondage is a delusion.

The solution of Vedānta is that we are not bound,

we are free already. Not only so, but to say or think that we are bound is dangerous; it is a mistake; it is self-hypnotism. As soon as you say, "I am bound," "I am weak," "I am helpless," woe unto you! You rivet one more chain upon yourself. Do not say it; do not think it. I have heard of a man who lived in a forest and used to repeat day and night, "Sivoham"—"I am the Blessed One"—and one day a tiger fell upon him and dragged him away to kill him. People on the other side of the river saw this and heard the voice, so long as voice remained in him, saying, "Śivoham" —even in the very jaws of the tiger. There have been many such men. There have been men who, while being cut to pieces, have blest their enemies. "I am He, I am He, and so art thou. I am pure and perfect, and so are all my enemies. You are He, and so am I." That is the position of strength. There are, no doubt, great and wonderful things in the religions of the dualists. Wonderful is the idea of the Personal God apart from nature, whom we worship and love. Sometimes this idea is very soothing. But, says Vedānta, that feeling, is something like the effect that comes from an opiate; it is not natural. It brings weakness in the long run, and what this world wants today more than it ever did before is strength. It is weakness, says Vedānta, that is the cause of all misery in this world. Weakness is the one cause of suffering. We become miserable because we are weak. We lie, steal, kill, and commit other crimes, because we are weak. We suffer because we are weak. We die because we are weak. Where there is nothing to weaken us, there is no death or sorrow. We are miserable through delusion.

Give up the delusion and the whole thing vanishes. It is plain and simple indeed. Through all these philosophical discussions and tremendous mental gymnastics we come to this one religious idea, the simplest in the whole world.

Monistic Vedānta is the simplest form in which you can put the truth. A great mistake was made in India and elsewhere, because people did not look at the ultimate principles, but only thought of the process, which is very intricate indeed. To many these tremendous philosophical and logical propositions were alarming. They thought that these things could not be made universal, could not be followed in everyday practical life, and that under the guise of such a philosophy much laxity of living would arise. But I do not believe at all that monistic ideas preached to the world will produce immorality and weakness. On the contrary, I have reason to believe that they are the only remedy there is. If this be the truth, why let people drink ditch-water when the stream of life is flowing by? If this be the truth, that they are all pure, why not at this moment teach it to the whole world? Why not teach it, with the voice of thunder, to every man that is born, to saints and sinners, men, women, and children, to the man on the throne and to the man sweeping the streets?

It appears to be a very big and a very great undertaking; to many it appears very startling. But that is because of superstition, nothing else. By eating all sorts of bad and indigestible food, or by starving ourselves, we have become incompetent to eat a good meal. We have listened to words of weakness from our

childhood. You hear people say that they do not believe
in ghosts; but at the same time, there are very few
who do not feel a little creepy sensation in the dark.
It is simply superstition. So with all religious superstitions. There are people in this country who, if I
told them there was no such being as the Devil, would
think all religion was gone. Many people have said to
me: "How can there be religion without a Devil? How
can there be religion without a God to direct us? How
can we live without being ruled by somebody? We like
to be so treated, because we have become used to it.
We are not happy until we feel we have been repri-
manded by somebody every day." The same superstition! But however terrible it may seem now, the
time will come when we shall look back, each one of
us, and smile at every one of those superstitions which
covered the pure and eternal Soul, and repeat with
gladness, with truth, and with strength: "I am free,
and was free, and always will be free."

This monistic idea will come out of Vedānta, and
it is the one idea that deserves to live. The scriptures
may perish tomorrow. Whether this idea first flashed
in the brains of Hebrews or of people living in the
Arctic regions, nobody cares. For this is the truth and
truth is eternal; and truth itself teaches that it is not
the special property of any individual or nation. Men,
animals, and gods are all common heirs to this one
truth. Let them all receive it. Why make life miserable?
Why let people fall into all sorts of superstitions? Not
only in this country, but in the land of its very birth,
if you tell people this truth they are frightened. They
say: "This idea is for sannyāsins, who give up the

world and live in forests; for them it is all right. But as for us poor householders, we must all have some sort of fear, we must have ceremonies," and so on. Dualistic ideas have ruled the world long enough, and this is the result. Why not make a new experiment? It may take ages for all minds to receive monism, but why not begin now? If we have told about it to twenty persons in our lives, we have done a great work.

There is one idea which often militates against it. It is this: It is all very well to say, "I am the Pure, the Blessed," but I cannot show it always in my life. That is true; the ideal is always very hard. But would it mend matters to go towards superstition? If we cannot get nectar, would it mend matters for us to drink poison? Would it be any help for us, because we cannot realize Truth immediately, to go into darkness and yield to weakness and superstition?

I have no objection to dualism in many of its forms. I like most of them, but I do have objections to every form of teaching which inculcates weakness. This is the one question that I put to every man, woman, or child who is in physical, mental, or spiritual training: "How do you feel? Are you any stronger?"—for I know it is Truth alone that gives strength. I know that Truth alone gives life, and nothing but approaching Reality will make us strong, and that none will reach Truth until he is strong. Any system, therefore, which weakens the mind, which makes one superstitious, makes one mope, makes one desire all sorts of wild impossibilities, mysteries, and superstitions, I do not like, because its effect is dangerous. Such systems never bring any good; such things create morbidity in the mind, make it weak, so weak that in the course of time it will be almost impossible to receive Truth or live up to it. Strength, therefore, is the one thing needful. Strength is the medicine for the world's disease. Strength is the medicine which the poor must have when tyrannized over by the rich. Strength is the medicine which the ignorant must have when oppressed by the learned; and it is the medicine which sinners must have when tyrannized over by other sinners. And nothing gives such strength as this idea of monism; nothing makes us so moral as this idea of monism; nothing makes us work so well, at our best and highest, as when all the responsibility is thrown upon ourselves.

I challenge every one of you. How will you behave if I put a little baby in your hands? Your life will be changed for the moment. Whatever you may be, you must become selfless for the time being. You will give up all your criminal ideas as soon as responsibility is thrown upon you; your whole character will change. So if the whole responsibility is thrown upon our own shoulders, we shall be at our highest and best. When we have nobody to grope towards, no Devil to lay our blame upon, no Personal God to carry our burdens, when we alone are responsible, then we shall rise to our highest and best. "I am responsible for my fate, I am the bringer of good unto myself, I am the bringer of evil. I am the Pure and Blessed One." We must reject all thoughts that assert the contrary. "I have neither death nor fear, I have neither caste nor creed, I have neither father nor mother nor birth, neither friend nor foe; for I am Existence, Knowledge, and

Bliss Absolute; I am the Blissful One, I am the Blissful One. I am not bound either by virtue or by vice, by happiness or by misery. Pilgrimages and books and ceremonials can never bind me. I have neither hunger nor thirst; the body is not mine, nor am I subject to the superstitions and decay that come to the body. I am Existence, Knowledge, and Bliss Absolute; I am the Blissful One, I am the Blissful One."

This, says Vedānta, is the only prayer that we should have. This is the only way to reach the goal: to tell ourselves and to tell everybody else that we are divine. As we go on repeating this, strength comes. He who falters at first will get stronger and stronger, and the voice will increase in volume until Truth takes possession of our hearts and courses through our veins and permeates our bodies. Delusion will vanish as the light becomes more and more effulgent, load after load of ignorance will vanish, and then will come a time when all else has disappeared and the Sun alone shines.

THE COSMOS

THE MACROCOSM

(Delivered in New York, January 19, 1896)

THE FLOWERS that we see all around us are beautiful, beautiful is the rising of the morning sun,
beautiful are the variegated hues of nature. The whole
universe is beautiful, and man has been enjoying it
since his appearance on earth. Sublime and awe-inspiring are the mountains, the gigantic rushing rivers rolling towards the sea, the trackless deserts, the infinite
ocean, the starry heavens; all these are awe-inspiring,
sublime, and beautiful indeed. The whole mass of
existence which we call nature has been acting on the
human mind from time immemorial. It has been acting on the thought of man, and as its reaction has
come the question: "What are these? Whence are
they?"

As far back as the time of the oldest portion of that
most ancient human composition, the Vedas, we find
the same question asked: "Whence is this? When there
was neither aught nor naught, and darkness was hidden in darkness, who projected this universe? How?
Who knows the secret?" And the question has come
down to us at the present time. Millions of attempts
have been made to answer it, yet millions of times it
will have to be answered again. It is not that each
answer was a failure; every answer to this question

contained a part of the truth, and this truth gathers strength as time rolls on. I will try to present before you the outline of the answer that I have gleaned from the ancient philosophers of India, in harmony with modern knowledge.

We find that in this oldest of questions a few points had been already solved. The first is that there was a time when there was "neither aught nor naught," when this world did not exist; when the planets and luminaries, our mother earth, with the seas and oceans, the rivers and mountains, cities and villages, human beings, animals, plants, and birds—all this infinite variety of creation—had no existence. Are we sure of that? We shall try to trace how this conclusion was arrived at.

What does man see around him? Take a little plant. He puts a seed in the ground and later he finds a plant peep out, lift itself slowly above the ground, and grow and grow till it becomes a gigantic tree. Then it dies, leaving only a seed. It completes the circle: it comes out of the seed, becomes the tree, and ends in the seed again. Look at a bird—how from the egg it springs, lives its life, and then dies, having produced other eggs, seeds of future birds. So with the animals; so with men. Everything in nature begins, as it were, from certain seeds, certain rudiments, certain fine forms, and becomes grosser and grosser, and develops, going on in that way for a certain time, and again goes back to that fine form and subsides.

The raindrop in which the beautiful sunbeam is playing was drawn in the form of vapour from the ocean, went far away into the air, and reached a region where it changed into water and dropped down in its present form—to be converted into vapour again. So with everything in nature by which we are surrounded. We know that the huge mountains are being worked upon by glaciers and rivers, which are slowly but surely pounding them and pulverizing them into sand, which drifts away into the ocean, where it settles down on its bed, layer after layer, becoming hard as rock, once more to be heaped up into mountains in the future. These, again, will be pounded and pulverized, and thus things go on. From sand rise these mountains; unto sand they go.

If it be true that nature is uniform throughout, if it be true—and so far no human experience has contradicted it—that the same method under which a small grain of sand is created works in creating the gigantic suns and stars and all this universe; if it be true that the whole of this universe is built on exactly the same plan as the atom; if it be true that the same law prevails throughout the universe, then if we take up a little plant and study its life, we shall know the universe as it is—as it has been said in the Vedas, "knowing one lump of clay, we know the nature of all the clay in the universe." If we know one grain of sand, we shall know the secret of the whole universe. Applying this type of reasoning to phenomena in general, we find, in the first place, that everything is similar at the beginning and the end. The mountain comes from sand and goes back to sand; the river comes out of vapour and goes back to vapour; plant life comes from the seed and goes back to the seed; human life comes out of the human germ and goes back to the germ. The universe with its stars and planets has come out of a nebulous state and must go back to it. And what do we learn from this? That the manifested or grosser state is the effect, and the finer state, the cause.

Thousands of years ago it was demonstrated by Kapila, the great father of philosophy, that destruction means going back to the cause. If this table here is destroyed it will go back to its cause, to those fine forms and particles which, combined, made this form which we call a table. If a man dies he will go back to the elements which gave him his body; if this earth dies it will go back to the elements which gave it form. This is what is called destruction: going back to the cause. Therefore we learn that the effect is the same as the cause, not different. It is only in another form. This glass is an effect, and it had its cause, and this cause is present in this form. A certain amount of the material called glass plus the force in the hands of the manufacturer are the causes, the material and the instrumental, which, combined, produced this form called a glass. The force which was in the hands of the manufacturer is present in the glass as the power of adhesion, without which the particles would fall apart; and the glass material is also present. The glass is only a manifestation of these fine causes in a new shape; and if it be broken to pieces the force which was present in the form of adhesion will go back and join its own element, and the particles of glass will remain the same until they take new forms. Thus we find that the effect is never different from the cause. It is only a reproduction of the cause in a grosser form.

Next we learn that all these particular forms, whether they are plants, animals, or men, are being repeated *ad infinitum,* rising and falling. The seed produces the tree; the tree produces the seed, which again comes up as another tree; and so on and on. There is no end to it. Water-drops roll down the mountains into the ocean and rise again as vapour, going back to the mountains and again coming down to the ocean. So, rising and falling, the cycle goes on.

So with all lives; so with all existence that we can see, feel, hear, or imagine. Everything that is within the bounds of our knowledge is proceeding in the same way, like breathing in and breathing out in the human body. Everything in creation goes on in this form, one wave rising, another falling, rising again, falling again. Each wave has its hollow; each hollow has its wave.

The same law must apply to the universe taken as a whole, because of its uniformity. This universe must be resolved into its causes; the sun, moon, stars, and earth, the body and mind, and everything in this universe, must return to their finer causes, disappear, be destroyed as it were. But they will live in the causes as fine forms. Out of these fine forms they will emerge again as new earths, suns, moons, and stars.

There is one fact more to learn about this rising and falling. The seed does not immediately become a tree, but has a period of inactivity, or rather, a period of very fine unmanifested action. The seed has to work for some time beneath the soil. It breaks into pieces, degenerates, as it were, and regeneration comes out of that degeneration. In the beginning the whole of this universe has to work likewise, for a period, in that subtle form, unseen and unmanifested, which is called chaos; and out of that comes a new projection. The whole period of one manifestation of this universe—its going back to the finer form, remaining there for some time, and coming out again—is, in Sanskrit, called a kalpa, or cycle.

Next comes a very important question, especially for modern times. We see that the finer forms develop slowly, and slowly and gradually become grosser and grosser. We have seen that the cause is the same as the effect, and the effect is only the cause in another form. Therefore this whole universe cannot have been produced out of nothing. There is nothing which is produced without a cause, and the cause is the effect in another form.

Out of what has this universe been produced, then? From a preceding fine universe. Out of what has man been produced? The preceding fine form. Out of what has the tree been produced? Out of the seed; the whole of the tree was there in the seed. It comes out and becomes manifest. So the whole of this universe has been created out of this very universe existing in a minute form. It has been made manifest now; it will go back to that minute form and again will be made manifest.

Now we find that the fine forms slowly come out and become grosser and grosser until they reach their limit, and when they reach their limit they go back farther and farther, becoming finer and finer again. This coming out of the fine and becoming gross, simply changing the arrangements of the parts, as it were, is in modern times called evolution. This is very true, perfectly true; we see it in our lives. No rational man can possibly quarrel with the evolutionists.

But we have to learn one thing more. We have to go one step farther. And what is that? That every evolution is preceded by an involution. The seed is the father of the tree, but another tree was itself the father of the seed. The seed is the fine form out of which the big tree comes, and that big tree was involved in that seed. The whole of this universe was present in the fine universe. The little cell which afterwards becomes the man is simply the man involved and becomes evolved as a man. If this is accepted, we have no quarrel with the evolutionists; for we see that if they admit this step, instead of destroying religion they will be its greatest supporters.

We see, then, that there is nothing that can be created out of nothing. Everything exists through eternity and will exist through eternity. Only the movement is in succeeding waves and hollows, going back to fine forms and coming out into gross manifestations. Involution and evolution are going on throughout the whole of nature. The whole series of evolution, beginning with the lowest manifestation of life and reaching up to the highest, the most perfect man, must have been the involution of something else. The question is, the involution of what? What was involved? God. The evolutionist will tell you that your idea that it was God is wrong. Why? Because, replies the evolutionist, you say that God is intelligent, but we find that intelligence develops much later in the course of evolution: it is in man and the higher animals that we find intelligence, but millions of years passed in this world before this intelligence was produced.

This objection of the evolutionists, however, does not hold water, as we shall see by applying our theory. The tree comes out of the seed, goes back to the seed; the beginning and the end are the same. The earth comes out of its cause and returns to it. We know that if we can find the beginning we can find the end. Conversely, if we find the end we can find the beginning. If that is so, take this whole evolutionary series, from the protoplasm at one end to the perfect man at the other. This whole series is one life. In the end we find perfection; so in the beginning there must have been the same. Therefore the protoplasm was the involution of the highest intelligence. You may not see it, but that involved intelligence is what is uncoiling itself until it becomes manifested in the most perfect man. And that can be mathematically demonstrated.

If the law of the conservation of energy is true, you cannot get anything out of a machine unless you first put it in. The amount of work you get out of an engine is exactly the same as the amount you have put into it in the form of water and coal—neither more nor less. The work I am doing now is just what I put into me in the shape of air, food, and other things. It is only a question of change and manifestation. There cannot be added in the economy of this universe one particle of matter or one foot-pound of force, nor can one particle of matter or one foot-pound of force be taken out. If that be so, what is this intelligence? If it was not present in the protoplasm,

it must have come all of a sudden, something coming
out of nothing, which is absurd. It therefore follows
absolutely that the perfect man, the free man, the
God-man, who has gone beyond the laws of nature
and transcended everything, who has no more to go
through this process of evolution, through birth and
death—that man called the "Christ-man" by the
Christians, the "Buddha-man" by the Buddhists, and
the "Free Soul" by the yogis—that perfect man who
is at one end of the chain of evolution was involved
in the protoplasmic cell, which is at the other end
of the same chain.

Applying the same sort of reasoning to the whole
of the universe, we see that intelligence must be the
lord of creation, the cause. What is the most evolved
notion that man has of this universe? It is that of
intelligence, the adjustment of part to part, the display
of intelligence—which notion the ancient design
theory attempted to express. The beginning is therefore intelligence. At the beginning that intelligence
becomes involved, and in the end that intelligence
becomes evolved. The sum total of the intelligence
displayed in the universe must therefore be the
involved universal intelligence unfolding itself. This
universal intelligence is what we call God. Call it by
any other name, it is absolutely certain that in the
beginning there is that infinite cosmic intelligence.
This cosmic intelligence gets involved, and it manifests,
evolves itself, until it becomes the perfect man, the
"Christ-man," the "Buddha-man." Then it goes back to
its own source. That is why all the scriptures say, "In
Him we live, and move, and have our being." That is

why all the scriptures preach that we come from God and go back to God. Do not be frightened by theological terms; if terms frighten you, you are not fit to be philosophers. This cosmic intelligence is what the theologians call God.

I have been asked many times, "Why do you use that old word *God*?" Because it is the best word for our purpose. You cannot find a better word than that, because all the hopes, aspirations, and happiness of humanity have been centred in that word. It is impossible now to change the word. Words like this were first coined by great saints, who realized their import and understood their meaning. But as they become current in society, ignorant people take up these words and the result is that they lose their spirit and glory. The word *God* has been used from time immemorial, and the idea of this cosmic intelligence and all that is great and holy is associated with it. Do you mean to say that because some fool says it is not all right, we should throw it away? Another man may come and say, "Take *my* word," and another, again, "Take *my* word." So there will be no end to foolish words. Use the old word, only use it in the true spirit, cleanse it of superstition, and realize fully what this great ancient word means. If you understand the power of the law of association, you will know that these words are associated with innumerable majestic and powerful ideas; they have been used and worshipped by millions of human souls and associated by them with all that is highest and best, all that is rational, all that is lovable, and all that is great and grand in human nature. And they suggest these associations and therefore cannot be given up.

If I had tried to express all this by telling you only that God created the universe, it would have conveyed nothing to you. Yet after all this struggle we have come back to Him, the Ancient and Supreme One.

We now see that all the various forms of cosmic energy, such as matter, thought, force, intelligence, and so forth, are simply the manifestation of that cosmic intelligence, or, as we shall call it henceforth, the Supreme Lord. Everything that you see, feel, or hear— the whole universe—is His creation, or to be a little more accurate, is His projection, or to be still more accurate, is the Lord Himself. It is He who is shining as the sun and the stars. He is mother earth; He Himself is the ocean. He comes as gentle showers, He is the gentle air that we breathe, and He it is who is working as force in the body. He is the speech that is uttered; He is the man who is talking. He is the audience that is here; He is the platform on which I stand; He is the light that enables me to see your faces. It is all He. He Himself is both the material and the efficient cause of this universe, and He it is that becomes involved in the minute cell and evolves at the other end and becomes God again. He it is that comes down and becomes the lowest atom, and slowly unfolding His nature, rejoins Himself.

This is the mystery of the universe. "Thou art the man, Thou art the woman, Thou art the strong man walking in the pride of youth, Thou art the old man tottering on crutches. Thou art in everything, Thou art everything, O Lord." This is the only solution of the cosmos that satisfies the human intellect. In one word, we are born of Him, we live in Him, and unto Him we return.

THE COSMOS

THE MICROCOSM

(Delivered in New York, January 26, 1896)

THE HUMAN MIND naturally wants to get outside, to peer out of the body, as it were, through the channels of the organs. The eye must see, the ear must hear, the senses must sense the external world; and naturally the beauties and sublimities of nature captivate the attention of man first. The first questions that arose in the human soul were about the external world. The solution of the mystery of the sky, of the stars, of the heavenly bodies, of the earth, of the rivers, of the mountains, of the ocean, was asked for; and in all ancient religions we find traces of how the groping human mind at first got hold of everything external. It believed in a river-god, a sky-god, a cloud-god, a rain-god; everything external, all that we now call the forces of nature, became metamorphosed, transfigured into gods, into heavenly powers.

As the inquiry went deeper and deeper, these external manifestations failed to satisfy the human mind, and finally it turned its energy inward and the question was asked about man's own soul. From the cosmos the question was reflected back to the microcosm; from the external world the question was reflected to the internal. From the analysing of external nature, man was led to the analysing of internal nature.

134

This questioning about the internal man comes with a higher state of civilization, with a deeper insight into nature, with a higher state of growth.

The subject of discussion this afternoon is the internal man. No question is so near and dear to man's heart as that of the internal man. How many millions of times, in how many countries, has this question been asked! Sages and kings, rich and poor, saints and sinners, every man, every woman, all have from time to time asked this question: Is there nothing permanent in this evanescent human life? Is there nothing, they have asked, which does not die when the body dies? Does not something endure when the physical frame crumbles into dust? Is there not something which survives the fire which burns the body into ashes? And if there is, what is its destiny? Where does it go? Whence did it come? These questions have been asked again and again, and so long as this creation lasts, so long as there are human brains to think, these questions will have to be asked.

Yet it is not that the answer did not come. Each time the question was raised the answer came; and as time rolls on, the answer will gain more and more strength. In fact the question was answered, once for all, thousands of years ago, and through all subsequent time that answer is being restated, reillustrated, made clearer to our intellect. What we have to do, therefore, is merely to make a restatement of the answer. We do not pretend to throw any new light on these all-absorbing problems, but we shall try to put before you the ancient truth in the language of modern times, to speak the thoughts of the ancients in the language

of the moderns, to speak the thoughts of the philosophers in the language of the people, to speak the
thoughts of the angels in the language of men, to
speak the thoughts of God in the language of poor
humanity, so that man will understand them; for the
same Divine Essence from which the ideas emanated
is ever present in man, and therefore he can always
understand them.

I am looking at you. How many things are necessary
for this vision? First, the eyes. For if I am perfect in
every other way, yet have no eyes, I shall not be able
to see you. Secondly, the real organ of vision. For the
eyes are not the organs; they are but the instruments
of vision, and behind them is the real organ, the
nerve-centre in the brain. If that centre be injured,
a man may have the clearest pair of eyes, yet he will
not be able to see anything. So it is necessary that
this centre, or the real organ, be there. Similarly, the
external ear is but the instrument for carrying the
vibration of sound inward to the centre. Thus with all
our senses. Yet that is not sufficient. Suppose in your
library you are intently reading a book, and the clock
strikes but you do not hear it. The sound is there, the
vibrations in the air are there, the ear and the centre
are also there, and these vibrations have been carried
through the ear to the centre, and yet you do not
hear it. What is wanting? The mind is not there. Thus
we see that the third thing necessary is that the mind
should be there. First there must be the external instrument, then the organ to which this external instrument will carry the sensation, and lastly the organ
itself must be joined to the mind. When the mind is

not joined to the organ, the organ and the ear may take the impression and yet we shall not be conscious of it. The mind, too, is only the carrier; it has to carry the sensation still farther and present it to the intellect. The intellect is the determinative faculty and decides upon what is brought to it. Still this is not sufficient. The intellect must carry it farther and present the whole thing before the ruler in the body, the human soul, the king on the throne. Before him this is presented, and then from him comes the order as to what to do or what not to do; and the order goes down, in the same sequence, to the intellect, to the mind, to the organs; and the organs convey it to the instruments, and perception is complete.

The instruments are in the external body, the gross body, of man; but the mind and the intellect are not. They are in what is called in Hindu philosophy the fine body, and what in Christian theology you read of as the spiritual body of man—finer, very much finer, than the body, and yet not the soul. The soul is beyond them all. The external body perishes in a few years; any simple cause may disturb and destroy it. The fine body does not perish so easily; yet it sometimes degenerates and at other times becomes strong. We see how, in an old man, the mind loses its strength, how, when the body is vigorous, the mind becomes vigorous, how various medicines and drugs affect it, how everything external acts on it, and how it reacts on the external world. Just as the body has its progress and decadence, so also has the mind, and therefore the mind is not the soul, because the soul can neither decay nor degenerate.

How can we know that? How can we know that
there is something behind this mind? Because knowledge, which is self-illuminating and the basis of intelligence, cannot belong to dull, dead matter. Never
was seen any gross matter which had intelligence as its
own essence. No dull or dead matter can illumine
itself. It is intelligence that illumines all matter. This
hall is known only through intelligence, because, as a
hall, its existence would be unknown unless some
intelligence perceived it. This body is not self-
luminous; if it were, it would be so in a dead man
also. Neither can the mind, nor even the spiritual
body, be self-luminous. They are not essentially
intelligent. That which is self-luminous cannot decay.
The luminosity of that which shines through a borrowed light comes and goes; but that which is light
itself—what can make that come and go, flourish and
decay? We see that the moon waxes and wanes because it shines through the borrowed light of the sun.
If a lump of iron is put into the fire and made red-
hot, it glows and shines; but its light will vanish
because it is borrowed. So decadence is possible only
of that light which is borrowed and is not light in its
own essence.

Now we see that the body, the external form, has
no light as its own essence, is not self-luminous, and
cannot know itself; neither can the mind. Why not?
Because the mind waxes and wanes; because it is
vigorous at one time and weak at another; because it
can be acted upon by anything and everything. Therefore the light which shines through the mind is not
its own. Whose is it, then? It must belong to That

which has light as Its own essence and, as such, can never decay or die, never become stronger or weaker—to the Soul, which is self-luminous, which is luminosity itself. It cannot be that the Soul knows; It *is* knowledge. It cannot be that the Soul has existence; It *is* existence. It cannot be that the Soul is happy; It *is* happiness. That which is happy has borrowed its happiness; that which has knowledge has received its knowledge; and that which has relative existence has only a reflected existence. Wherever there are qualities, these qualities have been reflected upon the substance. But the Soul does not have knowledge, existence, and blessedness as Its qualities; they are the essence of the Soul.

Again, it may be asked, why should we take this for granted? Why should we admit that the Soul has knowledge, blessedness, and existence as Its essence, and has not borrowed them? It may be argued: Why not say that the Soul's luminosity, the Soul's blessedness, the Soul's knowledge are borrowed in the same way as the luminosity of the body is borrowed from the mind? The fallacy of arguing in this way will be that there will be no limit. From whom were these borrowed? If we say from some other source, the same question will be asked again. So at last we shall have to come to one who is self-luminous. To simplify matters, then, the logical way is to stop where we get self-luminosity, and proceed no farther.

We see, then, that the human being is composed first of this external covering, the body; secondly, of the fine body, consisting of mind, intellect, and ego. Behind them is the real Soul of man. We have seen

that all the powers of the gross body are borrowed
from the mind, and the mind, the fine body, borrows
its powers and luminosity from the Soul standing
behind.

A great many questions now arise about the nature
of the Soul. If the existence of the Soul is admitted
on the basis of the argument that It is self-luminous,
that knowledge, existence, and blessedness are Its
essence, it naturally follows that this Soul cannot have
been created from nothing. A self-luminous existence,
independent of any other existence, could never have
non-existence for its cause. We have seen that even the
physical universe cannot have come from nothing,
not to speak of the Soul. It always existed. There was
never a time when It did not exist; because if the
Soul did not exist, where was time? Time is in the
Soul; when the Soul reflects Its powers on the mind
and the mind thinks, then time appears. When there
was no Soul, certainly there was no thought, and without thought there was no time. How can the Soul,
therefore, be said to be existing in time, when time
itself exists in the Soul? It has neither birth nor death,
but it is passing through all these various stages. It is
manifesting Itself slowly and gradually from lower to
higher, and so on. It is expressing Its own grandeur,
working through the mind on the body, and through
the body It is grasping the external world and understanding it. It takes up a body and uses it, and when
that body has failed and is used up, It takes another
body, and so on It goes.

Here comes a very interesting doctrine, that doctrine which is generally known as the reincarnation of

the soul. Sometimes people get frightened at the idea; and superstition is so strong that even thinking men believe that they are the outcome of nothing, and then, with the grandest logic, try to deduce the theory that although they have come out of zero, they will be eternal ever afterwards. Those that come out of zero will certainly have to go back to zero. Neither you nor I nor anyone present has come out of zero, nor will go back to zero. We have been existing eternally, and will exist, and there is no power under the sun, or above the sun, which can undo your or my existence or send us back to zero. Now, this idea of reincarnation is not only not a frightening idea, but most essential for the moral well-being of the human race. It is the only logical conclusion that thoughtful men can arrive at. If you are going to exist in eternity hereafter, it must be that you have existed through eternity in the past; it cannot be otherwise.

I will try to answer a few objections that are generally brought against the theory. Although many of you will think they are very silly objections, still we have to answer them; for sometimes we find that the most learned men are ready to advance the silliest ideas. Well has it been said that there never was an idea so absurd that it did not find philosophers to defend it.

The first objection is: Why do we not remember our past? But do we remember all our past in this life? How many of you remember what you did when you were babies? None of you remember your babyhood; and if upon memory depends your existence, then this argument proves that you did not exist as babies,

because you do not remember your babyhood. It is
simply unmitigated nonsense to say that our existence
depends on our remembering it. How can we remember our past life? That brain is gone, broken into
pieces, and a new brain has been manufactured. What
has come to this brain is the resultant, the sum total,
of the impressions acquired in our past, with which
the mind has come to inhabit the new body. I, as I
stand here, am the effect, the result, of all the infinite
past which is tacked on to me.

Such is the power of superstition that many of those
who deny the doctrine of reincarnation believe that
we are descended from monkeys. But they do not
have the courage to ask why we do not remember our
monkey life! When a great ancient sage, a seer or a
prophet of old who came face to face with Truth,
says something, these modern men stand up and say,
"Oh, he was a fool!" But just use another name—
Huxley or Tyndall—then it must be true, and they
take it for granted. In place of ancient superstitions
they have erected modern superstitions; in place of the
old popes of religion they have installed modern popes
of science.

So we see that this objection as to memory is not
valid; and that is about the only serious objection
raised against this theory.

Although we have seen that it is not necessary
for the acceptance of this theory that there should be
the memory of past lives, yet at the same time we
are in a position to assert that there are instances which
show that this memory does come, and that each one
of us will get back this memory at the time of liberation,

when we shall find that this world is but a dream. Then alone will you realize in the soul of your soul that you are but actors and the world is a stage; then alone will the idea of non-attachment come to you with the power of thunder; then all this thirst for enjoyment, this clinging to life and this world, will vanish for ever; then the mind will see as clear as daylight how many times all these existed for you—how many millions of times you had fathers and mothers, sons and daughters, husbands and wives, relatives and friends, wealth and power. They came and went. How many times you were on the very crest of the wave, and how many times you were down at the bottom of despair! When memory brings all these to you, then alone will you stand as a hero and smile when the world frowns upon you. Then alone will you stand up and say: "I care not even for thee, O Death! What terrors hast thou for me?" This will come to all.

Are there any arguments, any rational proofs, for the reincarnation of the soul? So far we have been giving the negative side, showing that the opposite arguments to disprove it are invalid. Are there any positive proofs? There are—and most valid ones, too. No other theory except that of reincarnation accounts for the wide divergence that we find between man and man in their power to acquire knowledge. First let us consider the process by means of which knowledge is acquired. Suppose I go into the street and see a dog. How do I know it is a dog? I refer it to my mind, and in my mind are groups of all my past experiences, arranged and pigeon-holed, as it were. As soon as a new impression comes, I take it up and refer it to some of the old pigeon-holes, and as soon as I find a group of the same impressions already existing, I place it in that group and I am satisfied. I know it is a dog because it coincides with impressions already there. And when I do not find the cognates of a new experience inside, I become dissatisfied. When, not finding the cognates of an impression, we become dissatisfied, this state of mind is called ignorance; but when, finding the cognates of an impression already existing, we become satisfied, this is called knowledge. When one apple fell, men became dissatisfied. Then gradually they found out a series of the same impressions, forming, as it were, a chain. What was the chain they found? That all apples fell. They called this gravitation.

Now, we see that without a fund of already existing experiences any new experience would be impossible, for there would be nothing to which to refer the new impression. So if, as some of the European philosophers think, a child came into the world with what they call a *tabula rasa*, such a child would never attain to any degree of intellectual power, because he would have nothing to which to refer his new experiences. We see that the power of acquiring knowledge varies in each individual, and this shows that each one of us has come with his own fund of knowledge. Knowledge can only be got in one way, the way of experience; there is no other way to know. If we have not had the experience in this life, we must have had it in other lives.

How is it that the fear of death is everywhere? A

little chicken is just out of the egg and an eagle comes, and the chicken flies in fear to its mother. There is an old explanation (I should hardly dignify it by such a name)—it is called instinct. What makes that little chicken just out of the egg afraid to die? How is it that as soon as a duckling hatched by a hen comes near water it jumps into it and swims? It never swam before nor saw anything swim. People call it instinct. It is a big word, but it leaves us where we were before.

Let us study this phenomenon of instinct. A child begins to play on the piano. At first she must pay attention to every key she is fingering, and as she goes on and on for months and years, the playing becomes almost involuntary, instinctive. What was first done with conscious will does not require later on an effort of the will. This is not yet a complete proof. One half remains, and that is that almost all the actions which are now instinctive can be brought under the control of the will. Each muscle of the body can be brought under control. This is perfectly well known. So the proof is complete, by this double method, that what we now call instinct is the degeneration of voluntary actions. Therefore if the analogy applies to the whole of creation, if all nature is uniform, then what is instinct in lower animals, as well as in men, must be the degeneration of will.

From the study of the macrocosm we discovered that each evolution presupposes an involution, and each involution an evolution. How is instinct explained in the light of this knowledge? What we call instinct is the result of voluntary action. Instinct in men or animals must therefore have been created by their previous voluntary actions. When we speak of voluntary actions, we admit previous experience. This previous experience thus creates instinct. The little chicken's fear of death, the duckling's taking to the water, and all the involuntary actions in the human being, which are the result of past experiences, have now become instinctive.

So far we have proceeded very clearly, and so far the latest science is with us. The latest scientific men are coming back to the ancient sages, and as far as they have done so there is no difficulty. They admit that each man and each animal is born with a fund of experience, and that all the instincts in the mind are the result of past experience. "But what," they ask, "is the use of saying that that experience belongs to the soul? Why not say it belongs to the body, and the body alone? Why not say it is hereditary transmission?" This is the last question. Why not say that all the experience with which I am born is the resultant of all the past experience of my ancestors? The sum total of the experience from the little protoplasm up to the highest human being is in me, but it has come from body to body in the course of hereditary transmission. Where will the difficulty be?

This question is very nice, and we admit some part of this hereditary transmission. How far? As far as furnishing the material of the body. We, by our past actions, are born in a certain body, and the suitable material for that body comes from the parents who have made themselves fit to have our soul as their offspring. But the simple hereditary theory takes for granted, without any proof, the most astonishing proposition: that mental experience can be recorded in matter, that mental experience can be involved in matter.

When I look at you, in the lake of my mind there is a wave. That wave subsides, but it remains in fine form, as an impression. We understand a physical impression's remaining in the body. But what proof is there for assuming that the mental impression can remain in the body, since the body goes to pieces? What carries it? Even granting that it is possible for each mental impression to remain in the body—that every impression, beginning from the first man down to my father, was in my father's body—how could it be transmitted to me? Through the bioplasmic cell? How could that happen? The father's body does not come to the child *in toto*. The same parents may have a number of children. Then, from this theory of hereditary transmission, where the impression and the impressed are one, because both are material, it rigorously follows that, by the birth of every child, the parents must lose a part of their own impressions, or, if the parents should transmit the whole of their impressions, then, after the birth of the first child, their minds would be a vacuum.

Again, if in the bioplasmic cell the infinite amount of impressions from all time have entered, where and how can they exist there? This is a most impossible position, and until these physiologists can prove how and where those impressions live in that cell, and what they mean by a mental impression's sleeping in the physical cell, their position cannot be taken for granted.

So far it is clear, then, that these impressions are in the mind, that the mind comes to take birth after birth and uses the material most proper for it, and that the mind which has made itself fit for only a particular kind of body will have to wait until it gets that material. This we understand. The theory then comes to this: There is hereditary transmission so far as furnishing the material to the soul is concerned. But the soul migrates and manufactures body after body; and each thought we think and each deed we do is stored in it in fine forms, ready to spring up again and take a new shape. When I look at you a wave rises in my mind. It goes down, as it were, and becomes finer and finer, but it does not die. It is ready to start up again as a wave in the shape of memory. So all these impressions are in my mind, and when I die the resultant force of them will be upon me. A ball is here, and each one of us takes a mallet in his hands and strikes the ball from all sides; the ball goes from point to point in the room, and when it reaches the door it flies out. What carries it out? The resultant of all these blows. That will give it its direction. So what directs the soul when the body dies? The resultant, the sum total, of all the works it has done, of all the thoughts it has thought. If the resultant is such that it has to manufacture a new body for further experience, it will go to those parents who are ready to supply it with suitable material for that body.

Thus from body to body it will go, sometimes to a heaven, and back again to earth, becoming a man or some lower animal. In this way it will go on until it has finished its experience and completed the circle.

It then knows its own nature, knows what it is, and its ignorance vanishes. Its powers become manifest; it becomes perfect. No more is there any necessity for the soul to work through physical bodies, nor is there any necessity for it to work through fine or mental bodies. It shines in its own light and is free—no more to be born, no more to die.

We shall not go now into the particulars of this. But I shall bring before you one more point with regard to this theory of reincarnation: It is the theory that advances the freedom of the human soul. It is the one theory that does not lay the blame for all our weakness upon somebody else, which is a common human failing. We do not look at our own faults. The eyes do not see themselves; they see the eyes of everybody else. We human beings are very slow to recognize our own weakness, our own faults, so long as we can lay the blame upon somebody else. Men in general lay all the blame on their fellow men, or, failing that, on God; or they conjure up a ghost called fate.

Where is fate and what is fate? We reap what we sow. We are the makers of our own fate. None else has the blame, none else the praise. The wind is blowing; those vessels whose sails are unfurled catch it and go forward on their way, but those which have their sails furled do not catch the wind. Is that the fault of the wind? Is it the fault of the merciful Father, whose wind of mercy is blowing without ceasing, day and night, whose mercy knows no decay—is it His fault that some of us are happy and some unhappy?

We make our own destiny. His sun shines for the weak as well as for the strong. His wind blows for

saint and sinner alike. He is the Lord of all, the Father
of all, merciful and impartial. Do you mean to say
that He, the Lord of Creation, looks upon the petty
things of our life in the same light as we do? What
a degenerate kind of God that would be! We are like
little puppies, making life-and-death struggles here
and foolishly thinking that even God Himself will take
them as seriously as we do. He knows what the
puppies' play means. Our attempts to lay the blame on
Him, making Him the punisher and the rewarder,
are only foolish. He neither punishes nor rewards any.
His infinite mercy is open to everyone—at all times, in
all places, under all conditions—unfailing, unswerv-
ing. Upon *us* depends how we utilize it. Blame neither
man nor God nor anyone in the world. When you
find yourselves suffering, blame yourselves and try
to do better. This is the only solution of the problem.

Those that blame others—and alas! their number
is increasing every day—are generally miserable souls,
with helpless brains, who have brought themselves
to that pass through their own mistakes. Though they
blame others, this does not alter their position. It does
not serve them in any way. This attempt to throw the
blame upon others only weakens them the more.
Therefore blame none for your own faults; stand upon
your own feet and take the whole responsibility upon
yourselves. Say: "This misery that I am suffering is
of my own doing, and that very thing proves that it
will have to be undone by me alone. That which I
created I can demolish; that which is created by someone else I shall never be able to destroy." Therefore
stand up, be bold, be strong. Take the whole respon-

sibility on your own shoulders and know that you are the creator of your own destiny.

All the strength and succour you want is within yourselves. Therefore make your own future. Let the dead past bury its dead. The infinite future is before you, and you must always remember that each word, thought, and deed lays up a store for you, and that as the bad thoughts and bad works are ready to spring upon you like tigers, so also there is the inspiring hope that the good thoughts and good deeds are ready with the power of a hundred thousand angels to defend you always and for ever.

IMMORTALITY

(Delivered in America)

WHAT QUESTION has been pondered a greater number of times, what idea has led men more to search the universe for an answer, what question is nearer and dearer to the human heart, what question is more inseparably connected with our existence, than this one, the immortality of the human soul? It has been the theme of poets and sages, of priests and prophets. Kings on the throne have discussed it; beggars in the street have dreamt of it. The best of humanity have approached it, and the worst of men have hoped for it. The interest in the theme has not died yet, nor will it die so long as human nature exists.

Various answers have been presented to the world by various minds. Thousands, again, in every period of history have given up the discussion. And yet the question remains fresh as ever. Often in the turmoil and struggle of our lives we seem to forget it; but suddenly someone dies—one, perhaps, whom we loved, one near and dear to our hearts, is snatched away from us—and the struggle, the din, and the turmoil of the world around us cease for a moment, and the soul asks the old question: "What after this? What becomes of the soul?"

All human knowledge proceeds out of experience; we cannot know anything except by experience. All our reasoning is based upon generalized experience;

all our knowledge is but harmonized experience. Looking around us, what do we find? A continuous change. The plant comes out of the seed, grows into the tree, completes the circle, and comes back to the seed. The animal is born, lives a certain time, dies, and completes the circle. So does man. The mountains slowly but surely crumble away, the rivers slowly but surely dry up, rain comes out of the sea and goes back to the sea. Everywhere circles are being completed—birth, growth, development, and decay following each other with mathematical precision. This is our everyday experience.

Inside it all, behind all this vast mass of what we call life, of millions of forms and shapes, millions upon millions of varieties, from the lowest atom to the highest spiritual man, we find existing a certain unity. Every day we find that the walls that were thought to divide one thing from another are being broken down. The one life, which is coming to be recognized by modern science as one substance, manifesting itself in different ways and in various forms, runs through all like a continuous chain, of which all these various forms represent the links, link after link, extending almost infinitely, but of the same one chain. This is what is called evolution. It is an old, old idea, as old as human society, only it is getting fresher and fresher as human knowledge progresses.

There is one thing more, which the ancients perceived, but which in modern times is not yet so clearly perceived, and that is involution. The seed becomes the plant; a grain of sand never becomes a plant. It is the father that becomes the child; a lump

of clay never becomes a child. From what does this
evolution come?—is the question. What was the seed?
It was the same as the tree. All the possibilities of a
future tree are in that seed; all the possibilities of a
future man are in the little baby; all the possibilities
of any future life are in the germ. What is this? The
ancient philosophers of India called it involution. We
find, then, that every evolution presupposes an involution. Nothing can be evolved which is not already
there.

Here again modern science comes to our help. You
know by mathematical reasoning that the sum total of
the energy that is displayed in the universe is the
same throughout. You cannot take away one atom of
matter or one foot-pound of force. You cannot add to
the universe one atom of matter or one foot-pound of
force. Evolution, as such, does not come out of zero.
Then where does it come from? From previous involution. The child is the man involved, and the man
is the child evolved. The seed is the tree involved, and
the tree is the seed evolved. All the possibilities of life
are in the germ.

The problem becomes a little clearer. Add to it the
first idea, that of the continuity of life. In all creatures,
from the lowest protoplasm to the most perfect human
being, there is really but one life. Just as in one lifetime we have so many various phases of expression, the
protoplasm developing into the baby, the child, the
young man, the old man, so from the protoplasm up
to the most perfect man we get one continuous life, one
chain. This is evolution. But we have seen that each
evolution presupposes an involution. The whole of

this life, which slowly manifests itself, evolves from the lowest protoplasm to the perfected human being, the incarnation of God on earth—the whole of this series is but one life, and the whole of this manifestation must have been involved in that very protoplasm. This whole series, ending in the God-man, was involved in it, and slowly came out, manifesting itself slowly, slowly, slowly. The perfect man must have been there in the germ state, in minute form. Therefore this one force, this whole chain, is the involution of that cosmic life which is everywhere. It is this one mass of intelligence which, from the protoplasm up to the most perfect man, is slowly and slowly uncoiling itself. Not that it grows. Take away all ideas of growth from your mind. With the idea of growth is associated something coming from outside, something extraneous, which would give the lie to the truth that the Infinite, which lies latent in every life, is independent of all external conditions. It can never grow; It is always there, and only manifests Itself.

The effect is the cause manifested. There is no essential difference between the effect and the cause. Take this glass, for instance. There was the material, and that material plus the will of the manufacturer made the glass; these two were its causes and are present in it. In what form? Adhesion. If the force were not here, each particle would fall away. What is the effect, then? It is the same as the cause, only taking a different form, a different composition. When the cause is changed and limited for a time, it becomes the effect. We must remember this. Applying it to our idea of life: The whole of the manifestation of this one series, from the protoplasm up to the most perfect man, must be the very same thing as cosmic life. First it got involved and became finer; and out of that fine something, which was the cause, it has gone on evolving, manifesting itself, and becoming grosser.

But the question of immortality is not yet settled. We have seen that everything in this universe is indestructible. There is nothing new; there will be nothing new. The same series of manifestations are presenting themselves alternately, as if on a wheel, coming up and going down. All motion in this universe is in the form of waves, successively rising and falling. Systems after systems are coming out of fine forms, evolving themselves, and taking grosser forms, again melting down, as it were, and going back to the fine forms. Again they rise out of the fine forms, evolving for a certain period and then slowly going back to the cause. So with all life. Each manifestation of life comes up and then goes down again. What goes down? The form. The form breaks to pieces, but it comes up again.

In one sense even bodies and forms are eternal. How? Suppose we take a number of dice and throw them, and they fall in this order: 6—5—3—4. We take the dice up and throw them again and again. There must be a time when the same number will come again; the same combination must come. Now each particle, each atom, that is in this universe, I take for such a die, and these are being thrown out and combined again and again. All these forms before you are one combination. Here are the forms of a glass, a table, a pitcher of water, and so forth. This is one combination; in time it will all break up. But there must come a time when exactly the same combination will have come again: you will be here and this form will be here, this subject will be talked on, and this pitcher will be here. An infinite number of times this has been repeated, and an infinite number of times this will be repeated. Thus, so far as the physical forms are concerned, what do we find? That even the combination of physical forms is eternally repeated.

A most interesting conclusion that follows from this theory is the explanation of facts such as these: Some of you, perhaps, have seen a man who can read the past life of others and foretell the future. How is it possible for anyone to see what the future will be, unless there is a regulated future? Effects of the past will recur in the future, and we see that it is so. You have seen the big Ferris wheel[1] in Chicago. The wheel revolves and the little carriages in the wheel come regularly one after another; one set of people gets into these, and after they have gone round the circle they get out and a fresh batch of people gets in. Each one of these batches is like one of these manifestations, from the lowest animal to the highest man. Nature is like the chain of the Ferris wheel, endless and infinite, and these little carriages are the bodies or forms, in which fresh batches of souls are riding, going up higher and higher until they become perfect and come out of the wheel. But the wheel goes

[1] The first Ferris wheel was erected for the Columbian Exposition at Chicago in 1893.

on. And so long as the bodies are in the wheel, it
can be absolutely and mathematically foretold where
they will go; but not so of the souls. Thus it is possible
to read the past and the future with precision.

We see, then, that there is a recurrence of the same
material phenomena at certain periods, and that the
same combinations have been taking place through
eternity. But that is not the immortality of the soul.
We have observed that no force can die; no matter
can be annihilated. What then becomes of the soul?
It goes on changing, back and forth, until it returns
to the source from which it came. There is no motion
in a straight line; everything moves in a circle. A
straight line, infinitely produced, becomes a circle. If
that is so, there cannot be eternal degeneration for
any soul. It cannot be. Everything must complete
the circle and come back to its source.

What are you and I and all these souls? In our discussion of evolution and involution, we have seen that
you and I must be part of the cosmic consciousness,
cosmic life, cosmic mind, which got involved, and that
we must complete the circle and go back to this cosmic
intelligence, which is God. This cosmic intelligence
is what people call the Lord, or God, or Christ, or
Buddha, or Brahman; what the materialists perceive
as force, and the agnostics, as the infinite, inexpres-
sible Beyond. And we are all parts of that.

This is the second idea. Yet this is not sufficient;
there will be still more doubts. It is all very well to
say that there is no destruction for any force. But all
the forces and forms that we see are combinations.
This form before us is a composition of several com-

ponent parts, and every force that we know is similarly composite. If you take the scientific idea of force, and call every force the sum total, the resultant, of several forces, what becomes of your individuality? Everything that is a compound must sooner or later go back to its component parts. Whatever in this universe is the result of the combination of matter or force must sooner or later go back to its components. Whatever is the result of certain causes must die, must be destroyed. It gets broken up, dispersed, and resolved back into its components.

The soul is not a force; neither is it thought. It is the manufacturer of thought, but not thought itself; it is the manufacturer of the body, but not the body. Why so? We see that the body cannot be the soul. Why not? Because it is not intelligent. A corpse is not intelligent, nor a piece of meat in a butcher's shop. What do we mean by intelligence? We mean reactive power. We want to go a little more deeply into this.

Here is a pitcher. I see it. How? Rays of light from the pitcher enter my eyes and make a picture in my retina, which is carried to the brain. Yet there is no vision. What the physiologists call the sensory nerves carry this impression inward. But up to this point there is no reaction. The nerve-centre in the brain carries the impression to the mind, and the mind reacts, and as soon as this reaction comes, the pitcher flashes before me.

Take a more commonplace example. Suppose you are listening to me intently, and a mosquito is sitting on the tip of your nose and giving you that pleasant

sensation which mosquitoes alone can give; but you
are so intent on hearing me that you do not feel the
mosquito at all. What has happened? The mosquito
has bitten a certain part of your skin, and certain
nerves are there. They have carried a certain sensation
to the brain, and the impression is there. But the mind,
being otherwise occupied, does not react. So you are
not aware of the presence of the mosquito.

When a new impression comes, if the mind does
not react we shall not be conscious of it; but when
the reaction comes we feel, we see, we hear, and so
forth. With this reaction comes illumination, as the
Sāmkhya philosophers call it. We see that the body
cannot illumine, because in the absence of attention
no sensation is possible.

Cases have been known where, under peculiar conditions, a man who had never learnt a particular
language was found able to speak it. Subsequent
inquiries proved that the man had, when a boy, lived
among people who spoke that language and the impressions were left in his brain. These impressions remained stored up there until through some cause the
mind reacted and illumination came; and then the
man was able to speak the language. This shows that
the mind alone is not sufficient, that the mind itself
is an instrument in the hands of someone else. The
boy's mind contained that language, yet he did not
know it; but later there came a time when he did.
It shows that there is someone besides the mind; and
when the man was a boy that someone did not use
the power, but when the boy grew up he took
advantage of it and used it.

First, here is the body; second, the mind, or instrument of thought; and third, behind this mind is the
Self of man. The Sanskrit word is Ātman. As modern
philosophers have identified thought with molecular
changes in the brain, they do not know how to explain
the case just mentioned, and generally deny it. The
mind is intimately connected with the brain, which
dies every time the body changes. The Self is the
illuminator, and the mind is the instrument in Its
hands, and through that instrument It gets hold of
the external instruments; and thus comes perception.
The external instruments get hold of the impressions
and carry them to the organs—for you must remember
always that the eyes and ears are only receivers; it is
the internal organs, the nerve-centres, that act. In
Sanskrit these centres are called indriyas. They carry
sensations to the mind, and the mind presents them
farther back to another state of the mind, which in
Sanskrit is called chitta, and there they are organized
into will; and all these present them to the King of
kings inside, the Ruler on his throne, the Self of
man. He then sees and gives his orders. Then the
mind immediately acts on the organs, and the organs
on the external body. The real Perceiver, the real
Ruler, the Governor, the Creator, the Manipulator of
all this, is the Self of man.

We see, then, that the Self of man is not the body,
neither is It thought. It cannot be a compound. Why
not? Because everything that is a compound can be
seen or imagined. That which we cannot imagine or
perceive, which we cannot bind together, is not force
or matter, cause or effect, and cannot be a com-

pound. The domain of compounds is only so far as our mental universe, our thought universe, extends; beyond this it does not exist. That is as far as law reigns, and if there is anything beyond law, it cannot be a compound at all.

The Self of man, being beyond the law of causation, is not a compound. It is ever free and is the Ruler of everything that is within law. It will never die, because death means going back to the component parts, and that which was never a compound can never die. It is sheer nonsense to say that It dies.

We are now treading on finer and finer ground, and some of you perhaps will be frightened. We have seen that this Self, being beyond the little universe of matter and force and thought, is a simple, uncompounded entity, and therefore It cannot die. That which does not die cannot live. For life and death are the obverse and reverse of the same coin. Life is another name for death; and death, for life. One particular mode of manifestation is what we call life; another particular mode of manifestation of the same thing is what we call death. When the wave rises to the top it is life, and when it falls into the hollow it is death. If anything is beyond death, naturally it must also be beyond life.

I must remind you of the first conclusion, that the Soul of man is part of the cosmic energy, which is God. We now find that It is beyond life and death. You were never born and you will never die. What is this birth and death that we see around us? This belongs to the body only, because the Soul is omnipresent. "How can that be?" you may ask. "So many

people are sitting here, and you say the Soul is omnipresent?" What is there, I ask, to limit anything that
is beyond law, beyond causation? This glass is limited;
it is not omnipresent, because the surrounding matter
forces it to take this form, does not allow it to expand.
It is conditioned by everything around it and is therefore limited. But that which is beyond law and has
nothing to act upon it—how can that be limited? It
must be omnipresent. You are everywhere in the
universe.

How is it, then, that I am born and I am going
to die, and all that? That is the talk of ignorance,
hallucination of the brain. You neither were born nor
will die. You neither have had birth nor will have
rebirth nor life nor death nor anything. What do you
mean by coming and going? All shallow nonsense!
You are everywhere. Then what is this coming and
going? It is the hallucination produced by the change
of the fine body, which you call the mind. That is
what is coming and going—just a little speck of cloud
passing before the sky. As it moves, it may create the
illusion that the sky moves. Sometimes you see a
cloud moving before the moon, and you think the
moon is moving. When you are in a train you think
the land is flying, or when you are in a boat you think
the water moves. In reality you are neither going nor
coming, you have not been born nor are you going
to be reborn; you are infinite, ever present, beyond
all causation, and ever free. How could there be
mortality when there was no birth? Such a question
is out of place; it is arrant nonsense.

To come to a logical conclusion we shall have to

take one step more. There is no half-way house. You are metaphysicians, and there is no crying quarter. If, then, we are beyond all law, we must be omniscient, ever blessed; all knowledge must be in us, and all power and blessedness. Certainly. You are the omniscient, omnipresent Being of the universe. But of such Beings can there be many? Can there be a hundred thousand millions of omnipresent Beings? Certainly not. Then what becomes of us all? You are only one; there is only one such Self, and that one Self is you. Standing behind this little nature is what we call the Soul. There is only one Being, one Existence—the Ever Blessed, the Omnipresent, the Omniscient, the Birthless, the Deathless. "Through His control the sky expands, through His control the air breathes, through His control the sun shines, and through His control all live. He is the Reality in nature, He is the Soul of your soul—nay more, you are He, you are one with Him."

Wherever there are two, there is fear, there is danger, there is conflict, there is strife. When it is all one, who is there to hate, who is there to struggle with? When it is all He, with whom can you fight? This explains the true nature of life; this explains the true nature of being. This is perfection, and this is God. As long as you see the many, you are under delusion. "In this world of many, he who sees the One, in this ever changing world, he who sees Him who never changes, as the Soul of his own soul, as his own Self—he is free, he is blessed, he has reached the goal."

Therefore know that thou art He; thou art the God of this universe—*Tat tvam asi*. All these various ideas that I am a man or a woman, or sick or healthy, or strong or weak, or that I hate or I love, or have a little power, are but hallucinations. Away with them! What makes you weak? What makes you fear? You are the sole Being in the universe. What frightens you?

Stand up, then, and be free. Know that every thought and word that weakens you in this world is the only evil that exists. Whatever makes men weak, makes men fear, is the only evil that should be shunned. What can frighten you? If the suns come down and the moons crumble into dust and systems after systems are hurled to annihilation, what is that to you? Stand as a rock; you are indestructible. You are the Self, the God of the universe. Say: "I am Existence Absolute, Bliss Absolute, Knowledge Absolute. I am He." And like a lion breaking its cage, break your chain and be free for ever. What frightens you? What holds you down? Only ignorance and delusion; nothing else can bind you. You are the Pure One, the Ever Blessed.

Silly fools tell you that you are sinners, and you sit down in a corner and weep. It is foolishness, wickedness, downright rascality to say that you are sinners! You are all God. See you not God and call Him man? Therefore, if you dare, stand on that, mould your whole life on that. If a man cuts your throat, do not say no, for you are cutting your own throat. When you help a poor man, do not feel the least pride. That is worship for you and not a cause for pride. Is not the whole universe you? Where is there anyone that is not you? You are the Soul of this universe. You are the sun, moon, and stars; it is you that are shining

everywhere. The whole universe is you. Whom are
you going to hate or fight? Know, then, that you are
He, and model your whole life accordingly. He who
knows this and models his life accordingly will no
more grovel in darkness.

THE ĀTMAN: ITS BONDAGE AND FREEDOM

(Delivered in America)

ACCORDING TO THE Advaita philosophy there is only one thing real in the universe, which it calls Brahman. Everything else is unreal, manifested and manufactured from Brahman by the power of māyā. To reach back to Brahman is our goal. We are, each one of us, that Brahman, that Reality, plus māyā. If we can get rid of this māyā, or ignorance, then we become what we really are. According to this philosophy, each man consists of three parts: the body, the internal organ or mind, and behind that, what is called the Ātman, the Self. The body is the external coating, and the mind is the internal coating, of the Ātman, who is the real perceiver, the real enjoyer, the real Being in the body, who works the body by means of the internal organ, or mind.

The Ātman is the only reality in the human body and is immaterial. Because It is immaterial, It cannot be a compound, and because It is not a compound, It does not obey the law of cause and effect; and so It is immortal. That which is immortal can have no beginning, because everything with a beginning must have an end. It also follows that it must be formless; there cannot be any form without matter. Further, everything that has form must have a beginning and an

167

end. We have none of us seen a form which had no beginning and will have no end.

A form comes out of a combination of force and matter. This chair has a peculiar form, that is to say, a certain quantity of matter is acted upon by a certain amount of force and made to assume a particular shape. The shape is the result of a combination of matter and force. The combination cannot be eternal; there must come to every combination a time when it will dissolve. So all forms have a beginning and an end. We know our body will perish; it had a beginning and it will have an end. But the Self, having no form, cannot have any beginning and end. It has existed for an infinite time.

Secondly, It must be all-pervading. It is only form that is conditioned and limited by space; that which is formless cannot be confined in space. So, according to Advaita Vedānta, the Self, the Ātman, in you, in me, in everyone, is omnipresent. You are as much in the sun now as in this earth, as much in England as in America. But when the Self acts through a particular mind and body, Its action is visible.

Each work we do, each thought we think, produces an impression, called in Sanskrit samskāra, upon the mind, and the sum total of these impressions becomes the tremendous thing called character. The character of a man is what he has created for himself; it is the result of the mental and physical actions that he has done in his life. The sum total of the samskāras is the power which gives a man his next direction after death. A man dies; the body falls away and goes back to the elements; but the samskāras remain, adhering to the mind, which, being made of fine material, does not dissolve, because the finer the material, the more persistent it is. But in the long run the mind also dissolves, and this dissolution of the mind is our goal.

In this connexion, the best illustration that comes to my mind is that of the whirlwind. Different currents of air coming from different directions meet, and at the meeting-point become united and go on rotating; as they rotate they form a column, drawing in dust, bits of paper, straw, and so forth, at one place, only to drop them at another; and thus they continue to rotate, raising and forming bodies out of the materials which are before them. Even so the forces called prāna in Sanskrit come together and form the body and the mind out of matter, and move on until the body falls, when they gather other materials to make another body; and when this falls, still another; and thus the process goes on.

Force cannot travel without matter. So when the body falls, the mind-stuff remains, prāna acting on it, and then it goes on to another point, raises up another whirl from fresh materials, and begins another motion; and so it travels from place to place until the force is all spent, and then it falls down, exhausted. So when the mind comes to an end, is broken to pieces entirely, without leaving any samskāra, we shall be entirely free; and until that time we are in bondage—until then the Ātman is covered by the whirl of the mind and imagines It is being taken from place to place. When the whirl falls down, the Ātman finds that It is all-pervading. It can go where It likes, is entirely free, and is able to manufacture any number of minds or bodies It likes. But until then It can go only with the whirl. This freedom is the goal towards which we are all moving.

Suppose there is a ball in this room, and we each have a mallet in our hands and begin to strike the ball, giving it hundreds of blows, driving it from point to point, until at last it flies out of the room. With what force and in what direction it will go out will be determined by the forces that have been acting upon it all through the room. All the different blows that have been given will have their effects. Each one of our actions, mental and physical, is such a blow, and the human mind is the ball which is being hit. We are being hit about this room of the world all the time, and our passage out of it is determined by the force of all these blows. In each case the speed and direction of the ball are determined by the hits it has received; so all our actions in this world will determine our future birth. Our present birth, therefore, is the result of our past.

Here is an example: Suppose I give you a chain in which a black link alternates with a white link, the two forming a unit, and the chain is without beginning and end. If I ask you about the nature of the chain, you will at first find it difficult to determine, the chain being infinite at both ends. But you will soon discover that this chain is an endless repetition of the unit of black and white links. If you know the nature of one of these units, you know the whole chain, because it is a perfect repetition. Likewise, all our lives—past, present, and future—form, as it were, an infinite chain, without beginning and without end, each unit of which is one life, with two ends: birth and death. What we are and what we do here in this life is being repeated again and again, with but little variation. So if we know this one unit of life, we shall know all the lives we shall have to pass through in this world. We see, therefore, that our present life in this world has been exactly determined by our previous lives, that is to say, by our own past actions.

Just as we go out of this world with the sum total of our present actions upon us, so we come into it with the sum total of our past actions upon us; that which takes us out is the very same thing which brings us in. What brings us in? Our past deeds. What takes us out? Our own deeds here. And so on and on we go. Like the caterpillar, which takes the thread from its own mouth and builds its cocoon, and at last finds itself caught inside the cocoon, we have bound ourselves by our own actions, we have thrown the network of our actions around ourselves. We have set the law of causation in motion and we find it hard to get out of its control. We have set the wheel in motion and we are being crushed under it. So this philosophy teaches us that we are uniformly being bound by our own actions, good or bad.

The Ātman never comes or goes, never is born or dies. It is nature that moves before the Ātman; and the reflection of this motion is on the Ātman and the Ātman ignorantly thinks that It is moving, and not nature. When the Ātman thinks thus, It is in bondage, but when It comes to find that It never moves, that It is omnipresent, then It is free. The Ātman in bondage is called jiva. Thus you see that when it is said that the Ātman comes and goes, it is said only figuratively. So the jiva, the bound soul, comes to higher or lower states. This is the well-known law of reincarnation, and this law binds all creation.

People in this country think it too horrible that man should become an animal. Why? Are the animals nothing? If we have a soul, so have they, and if they have none, neither have we. It is absurd to say that man alone has a soul, and the animals have none. I have seen men worse than animals.

The human soul has sojourned in lower and higher forms, migrating from one to another according to its samskāras, or impressions; but it is only in the highest form, as man, that it attains to freedom. The man-form is higher even than the god-form; of all forms it is the highest. Man is the highest being in creation because he alone attains to freedom.

All this universe was in Brahman, and it was, as it were, projected out of It and has been moving on, to go back to the source from which it was projected— like electricity, which comes out of the dynamo, completes the circuit, and returns to it. It is the same with the soul. Projected from Brahman, it passed through all sorts of vegetable and animal forms, and at last it is in man; and man is nearest to Brahman.

To go back to Brahman, from which we have been projected, is the great struggle of life. Whether people know it or not does not matter. In the universe, whatever motion or struggle we see—in minerals or plants or animals—is an effort to come back to the centre and be at rest. There was an equilibrium, and that has been destroyed, and all parts—all atoms and molecules

—are struggling to find their lost equilibrium again. In this struggle they are combining and re-forming, giving rise to all the wonderful phenomena of nature. All struggles and competitions in animal life, plant life, and everywhere else, all social struggles and wars, are but expressions of the eternal struggle to get back to that equilibrium.

This going from birth to death, this travelling, is what is called samsāra in Sanskrit, literally, the round of birth and death. All creation, passing through this round, will sooner or later become free. The question may be raised: If we all shall come to freedom, why should we *struggle* to attain it? If everyone is going to be free, why not sit down and wait? If it is true that every being will become free sooner or later and no one will be lost, that nothing will come to destruction and everything must be liberated—if that is so, what is the use of our struggling?

In the first place, the struggle is the only means that will bring us to the centre. And in the second place, we do not know why we struggle; we have to. "Of thousands of men, some are awakened to the idea that they must become free." The vast masses of mankind are content with material things; but there are some who are awake and want to get back, who have had enough of this playing here. These struggle consciously, while the rest do it unconsciously.

The alpha and omega of Vedānta philosophy is to give up the world, give up the unreal and take the real. Those who are enamoured of the world may ask: "Why should we attempt to get out of it, to go back to the centre? Suppose we have all come from

God; but we find this world is pleasurable and nice.
Then why should we not rather try to get more and
more from the world? Why should we try to get out
of it?" They say: "Look at the wonderful improvements going on in the world every day—how much
luxury is being manufactured for us! This is very
enjoyable; why should we go away and strive for
something which is not like this?"

The answer is that the world is impermanent and
changing, and many times we have had the same enjoyments. All the forms we are seeing now have been
manifested again and again, and the world in which
we live has been here many times before. I have been
here and talked to you many times before. You will
see that it must be so; and the very words that you
have been listening to now you have heard many
times before. And many times more it will be the
same. The souls were never different; only the bodies
have been constantly dissolving and recurring. Secondly, these things occur periodically. Suppose you
have three or four dice, and when you throw them,
one comes up five, another four, another three, and
another two. If you keep on throwing, there must
come times when those very same numbers will recur.
Go on throwing, and no matter how long may be the
interval, those numbers must come again. It cannot be
asserted when they will come again. This is determined by the law of chance. So with souls and their
associations. However distant may be the periods, the
same combinations and dissolutions will happen again
and again. The same birth, eating, and drinking, and
then death, come round again and again. Some never

find anything higher than the enjoyments of the world; but those who want to soar higher find that these enjoyments are never final, are only by the way.

Every form, let us say, beginning from the little worm and ending in man, is like one of the cars of the Ferris wheel. The car is in motion all the time, but the occupants change. A man gets into the car, moves with the wheel, and comes out. The wheel goes on and on. A soul enters one form, resides in it for a time, then leaves it and goes into another, and quits that again for a third. Thus it goes on, till it comes out of the wheel and becomes free.

Astonishing powers of reading the past and the future of a man's life have been known in every country and every age. The explanation is that so long as the Ātman is within the realm of causation, although its inherent freedom is not entirely lost and can assert itself even to the extent of taking the soul out of the causal chain—as it does in those men who become free—its actions are greatly influenced by the causal law and thus make it possible for men possessed of the insight to trace the sequence of effects, to tell the past and the future.

So long as there is desire or want, it is a sure sign that there is imperfection. A perfect, free being cannot have any desire. God cannot want anything. If He desired, He could not be God; He would be imperfect. So all the talk about God's desiring this and that, and becoming angry and pleased by turns, is babies' talk; it means nothing. Therefore it has been taught by all teachers: "Desire nothing. Give up all desires and be perfectly satisfied."

A child comes into the world crawling and without teeth, and the old man goes out crawling and without teeth. The extremes are alike, but the one has no experience of the life before him, while the other has gone through it all. When the vibrations of the ether are very low, we do not see light; there is darkness. When they are very high, the result is also darkness. The extremes generally appear to be the same, though the one is as distant from the other as the poles. The wall has no desires, and neither has the perfect man. But the wall is not sentient enough to desire, while for the perfect man there is nothing to desire. There are idiots who have no desires in this world, because their brains are imperfect. At the same time, the highest state is reached when we have no desires. But the two are opposite poles of the same existence: one is near to the animal, and the other near to God.

THE REAL AND THE APPARENT MAN

(Delivered in New York, February 16, 1896)

HERE WE STAND, and our eyes look forward, sometimes miles ahead. Man has been doing that since he began to think. He is always looking forward, looking ahead. He wants to know where he goes—even after the dissolution of his body. Various theories have been propounded, system after system has been brought forward, to suggest explanations. Some have been rejected, while others have been accepted, and thus it will go on so long as man is here, so long as man thinks. There is some truth in each of these systems. There is a good deal of what is not truth in all of them. I shall try to place before you the sum and substance, the result, of the inquiries in this line that have been made in India. I shall try to harmonize the various thoughts on the subject as they have come up from time to time among Indian philosophers. I shall try to harmonize the psychologists and the metaphysicians, and if possible, I shall harmonize them with modern scientific thinkers also.

The one theme of the Vedānta philosophy is the search after unity. The Hindu mind does not care for the particular; it is always searching after the general, nay, the universal. "What is that by knowing which everything else becomes known?"—that is the one theme. "As through the knowledge of one lump of clay all that is made of clay is known, similarly, what

177

is that by knowing which this whole universe will be known?"—that is the one search.

One part of this phenomenal universe, according to the Hindu philosophers, can be resolved into a material which they designate as ākāśa. All the things which are around us, and which we see, feel, touch, taste, are simply different manifestations of this ākāśa. It is all-pervading and fine. All that we call solids, liquids, or gases; figures, forms, or bodies; the earth, sun, moon, and stars—all these are composed of ākāśa.

What force is it which acts upon this ākāśa and manufactures this universe out of it? Along with ākāśa exists a universal energy. All forms of energy in the universe—all motion, attraction, nay, even thought— are but differing manifestations of that one energy which the Hindus call prāna. This prāna, acting on ākāśa, creates the whole of the universe. At the beginning of a cycle, prāna sleeps, as it were, in the infinite ocean of ākāśa. This ocean exists motionless in the beginning. Then arises motion in the ākāśa by the action of prāna; and as this prāna begins to move, to vibrate, out of this ocean come the various celestial systems—suns, moons, stars—the earth, human beings, animals, plants, and the manifestations of all the various forces and phenomena. Every manifestation of energy, therefore, according to the Hindus, is prāna. Every manifestation of matter is ākāśa.

When this cycle ends, all that we call solid will melt away into the next finer or the liquid form, that will melt into the gaseous, and that into finer and more uniform heat vibrations; and all will melt back into the original ākāśa. And what we now call attrac-

tion, repulsion, and motion will slowly resolve into
the original prāna. Then this prāna, it is said, will
sleep for a period, again to emerge and throw
out all these forms; and when this period ends, the
whole thing will subside again. Thus the process of
creation is going down and coming up, oscillating
backward and forward; in the language of modern
science, it becomes static during one period, and during another period it becomes dynamic. At one time it
remains potential, and at the next period it becomes
active. This alternation has gone on through eternity.

Yet this analysis is only partial. This much has been
known even to modern physical science. Beyond that
the research of physical science cannot reach. But the
inquiry does not therefore stop. We have not yet found
that one thing by the knowing of which everything
else is known. We have resolved the whole universe
into two components, into what are called matter and
energy, or what the ancient philosophers of India
called ākāśa and prāna. The next step is to resolve
ākāśa and prāna into their origin. Both can be resolved
into a still higher entity called mind. It is out of mind,
mahat, the universally existing thought-power, that
these two have been produced. Thought is a finer
manifestation than either ākāśa or prāna. It is thought
that splits itself into these two. The universal thought
existed in the beginning, and that manifested, changed,
evolved itself into these two: ākāśa and prāna. By the
combination of these two the whole universe has been
produced.

We next come to psychology. I am looking at you.
The external sensations are brought to me by the eyes;

they are carried by the sensory nerves to the brain.
The eyes are not the organs of vision; they are but the
external instruments; because if the real organ behind,
that which carries the sensation to the brain, is destroyed, though I may have twenty eyes I cannot see
you. The picture on the retina may be as complete as
possible, yet I shall not see you. Therefore the organ
is different from its instruments; behind the instruments, the eyes, there must be the organ. So it is with
all the sensations. The nose is but the instrument of
smell, and behind it is the organ. With every sense
we have, there is first the external instrument in the
physical body and behind that, in the same physical
body, there is the organ. Yet these are not sufficient.

Suppose I am talking to you, and you are listening
to me with close attention. Something happens, say a
bell rings; you will not, perhaps, hear the bell ring.
The vibrations of that sound come to your ear, strike
the tympanum, and the impression is carried by the
nerve to the brain; if the whole process is completed
when the impression is carried to the brain, why then
do you not hear? Something else is wanting: the mind
is not attached to the organ. When the mind detaches
itself from the organ, the organ may bring any news
to it, but the mind will not receive it. When it attaches
itself to the organ, then alone is it possible for the
mind to receive the news.

Yet even that does not explain perception. The
instruments may bring the sensation from outside, the
organs may carry it inside, the mind may attach itself
to the organ, and yet the perception may not be complete. One more factor is necessary: there must be a

reaction within. With this reaction comes knowledge. That which is outside sends, as it were, the current of news into my brain. My mind takes it up and presents it to the intellect, which groups it in relation to pre-received impressions and sends a current of reaction; and with that reaction comes perception. Here, then, is the intellect. The state of mind which reacts is called the buddhi, the intellect. Yet even this does not complete the process. One step more is required.

Suppose that here is a camera[1] and there a sheet of cloth, and I want to throw a picture on that sheet. What must I do? I must guide various rays of light from the camera to fall upon the sheet and be focused there. Something that does not move is needed upon which to throw the picture. I cannot form a picture upon something which is moving; that something must be stationary, because the rays of light which I throw on it are moving, and these moving rays of light must be gathered, unified, co-ordinated, and completed, upon something stationary. So it is with the sensations which these organs of ours are carrying inside and presenting to the mind, and which the mind in its turn is presenting to the intellect. This process will not be completed unless there is something permanent in the background, upon which the picture, as it were, may be formed, upon which we may unify all the different impressions.

What is it that gives unity to the many changes of our being? What is it that keeps up the identity of the thing called individuality, moving from moment to moment? What is it by which all our different impres-

[1] Perhaps the Swami refers to a magic lantern.

sions are pieced together, and where the perceptions, as it were, come together, blend, and form a united whole? We have seen that there must be something to serve this end, and we also know that, relative to the body and mind, that something must be motionless. The sheet of cloth upon which the camera throws the picture is, relative to the rays of light, motionless; else there will be no picture. That is to say, the perceiver must be an individual. This something upon which the mind is painting all these pictures, this something upon which our sensations, carried by the mind and intellect, are placed and grouped and formed into a unity, is what is called the soul of man.

We have seen that it is the universal cosmic mind that splits itself into ākāśa and prāna, and beyond this mind we have found the soul in us. In the universe, behind the universal mind, there is also a Soul, and it is called God. In the individual it is the soul of man. In this universe, in the cosmos, just as the universal mind becomes evolved into ākāśa and prāna, even so we find that the Universal Soul Itself becomes evolved as mind. Is it really so with the individual man? Is his mind the creator of his body, and his soul the creator of his mind? That is to say, are his body, his mind, and his soul three different existences, or are they three in one, or are they different states of existence of one and the same entity? We shall try to find an answer to these questions.

The first step that we have now gained is this. Here is this external body; behind this external body are the organs, the mind, the intellect; and behind these is the soul. At the first step we have found, as it were, that the soul is separate from the body, separate from the mind itself. Opinions in the religious world become divided at this point, and the division is this: All those religious views which generally pass under the name of dualism hold that the soul is conditioned; that it has various qualities; that all feelings of enjoyment, pleasure, and pain really belong to the soul. The non-dualists deny that the soul has any such qualities; they say it is unconditioned.

Let me first take up the dualists and try to present to you their position with regard to the soul and its destiny; next, the system that contradicts them; and lastly, let us try to find the harmony which non-dualism will bring us.

This soul of man, because it is separate from the mind and body, because it is not composed of ākāśa and prāna, must be immortal. Why? What do we mean by mortality? Decomposition. And that is only possible for things that are the result of composition. Anything that is made of two or three ingredients must become decomposed. That alone which is not the result of composition can never become decomposed and therefore can never die. It must be immortal. It must have existed throughout eternity. It must be uncreate. Every item of creation is simply a composition; no one ever saw creation come out of nothing. All that we know of creation is the combination of already existing things into newer forms. That being so, the soul of man, being simple, must have been existing for ever, and must go on existing for ever.

When this body falls off, the soul lives on. According to the dualists, when the body dissolves, the

vital forces of the man go back to his mind and the
mind becomes dissolved, as it were, into the prāna,
and that prāna enters into the soul of man, and the
soul of man comes out, clothed with what they call
the fine body, the mental body, or the spiritual body,
as you may prefer to call it.

In this body lie the samskāras of the man. What
are the samskāras? This mind is like a lake, and every
thought is like a wave upon that lake. Just as, in a
lake, waves rise and then fall and disappear, so these
thought-waves are continually rising in the mind-stuff
and then disappearing. But they do not disappear for
ever. They become finer and finer, but they are all
there, ready to start up at another time, when called
upon to do so. Memory is simply the calling back into
wave-form of some of those thoughts which have gone
into that finer state of existence. Thus everything that
we have thought, every action that we have done, is
lodged in the mind; it is all there in fine form; and
when a man dies, the sum total of these impressions
use the fine body as a medium. The soul, clothed, as
it were, with these impressions and the fine body,
passes out, and its destiny is guided by the resultant of
all the different forces represented by the different
impressions.

According to the dualists there are three different
goals for the soul. Those who are very spiritual, when
they die follow the solar rays and reach what is called
the solar sphere; through that they reach what is called
the lunar sphere; and through that they reach what
is called the sphere of lightning. There they meet
with another soul, who is already blessed, and he

guides the new-comers forward to the highest of all spheres, which is called Brahmaloka, the sphere of Brahmā. There these souls attain to omniscience and omnipotence, become almost as powerful and all-knowing as God Himself; and they reside there for ever, according to the dualists; or, according to the non-dualists, they become one with the Universal Soul at the end of the cycle.

The next class of persons, those who have been doing good work with selfish motives, are carried by the results of their good works, when they die, to what is called the lunar sphere, where there are various heavens, and there they acquire fine bodies, the bodies of gods. They become gods and live there and enjoy the blessings of heaven for a long period; and after that period is finished, the old karma again begins to function and so they fall back to the earth. They come down through the spheres of air and clouds, and all these various regions, and at last reach the earth through raindrops. There on the earth they enter into some cereal, which is eventually eaten by men who are fit to supply them with material to make new bodies.

The last class, namely, the wicked, when they die become ghosts or demons and live somewhere midway between the lunar sphere and this earth. Some of these try to disturb mankind; others are friendly. After living there for some time they also fall back to the earth and become animals. After living for some time in animal bodies they are released and come back again as men, and thus get another chance to work out their salvation.

We see, then, that those who have nearly attained
to perfection, in whom only very little of impurity
remains, go to Brahmaloka through the rays of the
sun. Those, again, who were a middling sort of people,
who did some good work here with the idea of going
to heaven, go to the lunar sphere and there obtain
god-bodies; but they have again to become men in
order to have another chance to become perfect. And
those who are very wicked become ghosts and demons,
and then they may have to become animals; after that
they become men again and get another chance to
perfect themselves.

This earth is called the karma-bhumi, the sphere of
karma. Here alone man performs good or bad karma.
When a man wants to go to heaven, and does good
works for that purpose, he becomes a god and, as such,
does not store up any fresh karma. He just enjoys the
effects of the good works he did on earth; and when
this good karma is exhausted, there comes upon him
the resultant force of all the evil karma he had previously stored up in life, and that brings him down
again to this earth. In the same way, those who become ghosts remain in that state without giving rise
to fresh karma, but suffering the evil results of their
past misdeeds, and later on remain for a time in
animal bodies without storing up any fresh karma.
When that period is over, they too become men again.
The states of reward and punishment due to good and
bad karma have no power to generate fresh karma;
they are only to be enjoyed or suffered.

If there is an extraordinarily good or an extraordinarily evil karma, it bears fruit very quickly. For

instance, if a man who has been doing many evil things all his life, does one very good act, the result of that act will immediately appear; and when that result has been reaped, the evil acts are ready to produce their results also. All men who do certain good and great acts, but the general tenor of whose lives has not been correct, will become gods, and after living for some time in god-bodies, enjoying the powers of gods, will again have to become men. When the effect of the good acts is thus finished, the old evil karma comes up to be worked out. Those who do extraordinarily evil acts have to put on ghost-bodies and devil-bodies, and when the effect of those evil actions is exhausted, the little of good action which remains stored up in them makes them again become men.

The way to Brahmaloka, from which there is no more fall or return, is called the Devayāna, the Way of the Gods; the way to heaven is known as the Pitriyāna, the Way of the Fathers.

Man, therefore, according to dualistic Vedānta, is the greatest being in the universe, and this earth the best place in it, because only here is the greatest and the best chance for him to become perfect. Angels or gods, or whatever you may call them, all have to become men if they want to become perfect. This is the great centre, the wonderful opportunity—this human life.

We come next to another school of philosophy. There are Buddhists who deny the whole theory of the soul that I have just now been propounding. "What use is it," says the Buddhist, "to assume something as the substratum, as the background, of this

body and mind? Why may we not allow thought to
function? Why admit a third substance, beyond this
organism composed of mind and body—a third substance called the soul? What is its use? Is not this
organism sufficient to explain itself? Why take a new,
a third something?" These arguments are very powerful. This reasoning is very strong. So far as outside
research goes, we see that this organism is a sufficient
explanation of itself; at least, many of us see it in that
light. Why, then, need there be a soul as substratum,
a something which is neither mind nor body but stands
as a background for both mind and body? Let there
be only mind and body. Body is the name of a stream
of matter continuously changing. Mind is the name of
a stream of consciousness or thought similarly changing. How does one explain the apparent unity in the
body and the mind? This unity does not really exist.
Take, for instance, a lighted torch. If you whirl it
rapidly, you see a circle of fire. The circle does not
really exist, but because the torch is continually moving, it creates the appearance of a circle. So there is
no unity in this body; it is a mass of matter continually
rushing on, and this stream of matter you may call
one unity, if you like. So it is with the mind. Each
thought is separate from every other thought; it is
only the rushing current that leaves behind the illusion of unity; there is no need of a third substance.
This universal phenomenon of body and mind is all
that really is; do not posit something behind it.

You will find that this Buddhist thought has been
taken up by certain sects and schools in modern times,
and all of them claim that it is new—their own

invention. This has been the central idea of most of the Buddhist philosophies: that this world is itself all-sufficient; that you need not ask for any background at all. All that is, is this sense universe; what is the use of thinking of something as a support for this universe? Everything is the aggregate of qualities; why should there be a hypothetical substance in which they inhere? The idea of substance comes from the rapid succession of qualities, not from something unchangeable which exists behind them.

We see how wonderful some of these arguments are; and they appeal easily to the ordinary experience of men. In fact, not one in a million can think of anything other than phenomena. To the vast majority of men nature appears to be only a whirling, combining, mingling mass of change. Few of us ever have a glimpse of the calm sea behind. For us it is always lashed into waves; this universe appears to us only as a tossing mass of waves.

Thus we find these two opinions: One is that there is something behind both body and mind which is an unchangeable and immovable substance; and the other is that there is no such thing as immovability or unchangeability in the universe; it is all change and nothing but change.

The solution of this difference comes in the next step of thought, namely, the non-dualistic. It says that the dualists are right in finding something behind all as a background which does not change; we cannot conceive change without there being something unchangeable. We can only conceive something changeable by knowing something which is less changeable,

and this also must appear more changeable in comparison with something else which is less changeable;
and so on and on, until we are bound to admit that
there must be something which never changes at all.
The whole of this manifestation must have been
in a state of non-manifestation, calm and silent, being
the balance of opposing forces, so to say, when no force
operated, because force acts when a disturbance of
the equilibrium comes in. This universe is ever hurry-
ing on to return to that state of equilibrium again. If
we are certain of any fact whatsoever, we are certain of
this. When the dualists claim that there is something
which does not change, they are perfectly right; but
their analysis that it is something which is neither the
body nor the mind, something separate from them
both but underlying them, is wrong. Again, so far as
the Buddhists say that the whole universe is a mass
of change, they are perfectly right; for, so long as I am
separate from the universe, so long as I stand back and
look at something before me, so long as there are two
things, the looker-on and the thing looked upon, it
will appear always that the universe is one of change,
that it is continuously changing. But the truth of the
matter is that there are both change and changelessness
in this universe. It is not true that the soul and the
mind and the body are three separate existences. It is
the same thing which appears as the body, as the
mind, and as the thing beyond mind and body; but
it is not at the same time all these. He who sees the
body does not even see the mind; he who sees the
mind does not see that which he calls the soul; and
he who sees the soul—for him the body and mind

have vanished. He who sees only motion never sees absolute calm, and he who sees absolute calm—for him motion has vanished. A rope is taken for a snake. He who sees the rope as the snake—for him the rope has vanished; and when the delusion ceases and he looks at the rope, the snake has vanished.

There is, then, but one all-comprehending Existence, and that Existence appears as manifold. This Self, or Soul, or Substance, is all that exists in the universe. This Self, or Soul, or Substance, is, in the language of non-dualism, Brahman, and It appears to be manifold by the interposition of name and form. Look at the waves in the sea. Not one wave is really different from the sea; but what makes the wave apparently different? Name and form—the form of the wave and the name which we give to it: "wave." That is what makes it different from the sea. When name and form go, it is the same sea. Who can find any real difference between the wave and the sea? So this whole universe is that one Existence; name and form have created all these various differences.

When the sun shines upon millions of globules of water, upon each particle is seen a most perfect representation of the sun. So the one Soul, the one Self, the one Existence of the universe, being reflected on all these numerous globules of varying names and forms, appears to be various; but It is in reality only one. There is no "I" or "you"; it is all one. It is either all "I" or all "you." This idea of duality, of two, is entirely false, and the whole universe, as we ordinarily know it, is the result of this false knowledge. When discrimination comes, and man finds there are

not two but one, he finds that he is himself this
universe. It is I who am this universe as it now exists,
a continuous mass of change. It is I who am beyond
all changes, beyond all qualities, eternally perfect,
eternally blessed.

There is, therefore, but one Ātman, one Self,
eternally pure, eternally perfect, unchangeable, un-
changed. It has never changed. And all these various
changes in the universe are but appearances in that
one Self.

Upon It name and form have painted all these
dreams; it is the form that makes the wave different
from the sea. Suppose the wave subsides; will the form
remain? No; it will vanish. The existence of the wave
was entirely dependent upon the existence of the
sea, but the existence of the sea was not at all dependent upon the existence of the wave. The form remains
so long as the wave remains; but as soon as the wave
leaves it, the form vanishes; it cannot remain.

Name and form are the outcome of what is called
māyā. It is this māyā that creates individuals, making
one appear different from another. Yet it has no
existence. Māyā cannot be said to exist. Form cannot
be said to exist, because it depends upon the existence
of another thing. At the same time, it cannot be said
not to exist, seeing that it makes all this difference.
According to the Advaita philosophy, then, this māyā
or ignorance—or name and form; or, as it has been
called in Europe, "time, space, and causality"—is
showing us, out of this one Infinite Existence, the
manifoldness of the universe. As substance this universe is one. So long as a man thinks that there are

two ultimate realities, he is mistaken. When he has come to know that there is but one, he is right.

This is being proved to us every day—on the physical plane, on the mental plane, and also on the spiritual plane. Today it has been demonstrated that you and I, the sun, the moon, and the stars are but the different names of different spots in the same ocean of matter, and that this matter is continuously changing in its configuration. The particle of matter that was in the sun several months ago may be in the human being now; tomorrow it may be in an animal; the day after tomorrow it may be in a plant. It is ever coming and going. It is all one unbroken, infinite mass of matter, merely differentiated by names and forms. One point is called the sun; another, the moon; another, the stars; another, a man; another, an animal; another, a plant—and so on. And all these names are fictitious; they have no reality, because the whole is a continuously changing mass of matter. This very same universe, from another standpoint, is an ocean of thought, where each one of us is a point called a particular mind. You are a mind, I am a mind, everyone is a mind. And the very same universe viewed from the standpoint of Knowledge, when the eyes have been cleared of delusions, when the mind has become pure, appears as the unbroken Absolute Being, ever pure, unchangeable, immortal.

What, then, becomes of all this threefold eschatology of the dualist—that when a man dies he goes to heaven, or goes to this or that sphere, and that wicked persons become ghosts or animals, and so forth? None comes and none goes, says the non-dualist. How can

you come and go? You are infinite; where is the
place for you to go?

In a certain school a number of little children were
being examined. The examiner had foolishly put all
sorts of difficult questions to the little children. Among
others there was this question: "Why does the earth
not fall?" His intention was to bring out the idea of
gravitation or some other intricate scientific truth
from these children. Most of them could not even
understand the question, and so they gave all sorts of
wrong answers. But one bright little girl answered it
with another question: "Where should it fall?" The
very question of the examiner was nonsense on the
face of it. There is no up and down in the universe;
the idea is only relative. So it is with regard to the
Soul: the very question of birth and death in regard to
It is utter nonsense. Who goes and who comes? Where
are you not? Where is the heaven that you are not in
already? Omnipresent is the Self of man. Where is It
to go? Where is It not to go? It is everywhere. So all
this childish dream, this puerile illusion of birth
and death, of heavens and higher heavens, and of
lower worlds, all vanishes immediately for the perfect;
and for the nearly perfect it vanishes after showing
them the several scenes up to Brahmaloka. It continues
for the ignorant.

How is it that the whole world believes in going
to heaven and in dying and being born? I am studying
a book; page after page is being read and turned over.
Another page comes and is turned over. Who changes?
Who comes and goes? Not I, but the book. The whole
of nature is a book before the Soul. Chapter after

chapter is being read and turned over, and every now and then a scene opens. That is read and turned over; a fresh one comes; but the Soul is ever the same— eternal. It is nature that is changing, not the Soul of man. This never changes. Birth and death are in nature, not in you. Yet the ignorant are deluded: just as we think, under delusion, that the sun is moving, and not the earth, in exactly the same way we think that we are dying, and not nature. These are all, therefore, hallucinations. Just as it is a hallucination when we think that the fields are moving and not the railway train, exactly in the same manner are birth and death a hallucination.

When men are in a certain frame of mind, they see this very existence as the earth, the sun, the moon, the stars; and all those who are in the same state of mind see the same things. Between you and me there may be millions of beings on different planes of existence. They will never see us, nor we them; we see only those who are in the same state of mind and on the same plane with us. Those musical instruments respond which have the same attunement of vibration, as it were. If the state of vibration which may be called the "man-vibration" should be changed, no longer would men be seen here; the whole man-universe would vanish, and instead of that, other scenery would come before us, perhaps gods and the god-universe, or perhaps, for the wicked man, devils and the diabolic world. But all would be only different views of the one universe. It is this universe which, from the human plane, is seen as the earth, the sun, the moon, the stars, and all such things. It is this very universe which, seen from the plane of wickedness, appears as a place of punishment; and this very universe is seen as heaven by those who want to see it as heaven. Those who have been dreaming of going to a God who is sitting on a throne, and of standing there praising Him all their lives, when they die will merely see a vision of what they have in their minds. This very universe will simply change into a vast heaven, with all sorts of winged beings flying about, and a God sitting on a throne. These heavens are all of man's own making.

So what the dualist believes is true, says the non-dualist, but it is all simply of his own making. These spheres and devils and gods and reincarnations and transmigrations are all mythology. So also is this human life. The great mistake that men always make is to think that this life alone is real; they understand it well enough when other things are called mythologies, but are never willing to admit the same of their own position. The whole thing as it appears is mere mythology, and the greatest of all lies is to say that we are bodies, which we never were nor ever can be. It is the greatest of all lies to say that we are mere men. We are the God of the universe. In worshipping God we have always been worshipping our own hidden Self. The worst lie that you can ever tell yourself is that you were born a sinner or a wicked man. He alone is a sinner who sees a sinner in another man. Suppose there is a baby here, and you place a bag of gold on the table, and then a robber comes and takes the gold away. To the baby it is all the same: because there is no robber inside, he sees no robber outside.

To sinners and vile men there is vileness outside; but not to good men. So the wicked see this universe as hell, and the partially good see it as heaven, while perfect beings realize it as God Himself. Only when a man sees this universe as God does the veil fall from his eyes; then that man, purified and cleansed, finds his whole vision changed. The bad dreams that have been torturing him for millions of years all vanish, and he who had thought of himself as either a man or a god or a demon, he who had thought of himself as living in low places, in high places, on earth, in heaven, and so on, finds that he is really omnipresent; that all time is in him, and he is not in time; that all the heavens are in him, and he is not in any heaven; that all the gods that man ever worshipped are in him, and he is not in any one of those gods. He was the manufacturer of gods and demons, of men and plants and animals and stones. And the real nature of man now stands unfolded to him as being higher than heaven, more perfect than this universe of ours, more infinite than infinite time, more omnipresent than the omnipresent ether.

Thus alone does a man become fearless and free. Then all delusions cease, all fears come to an end for ever. Birth goes away and with it death; pains fly and with them fly away pleasures; earth vanishes and with it vanishes heaven; the body vanishes and with it vanishes the mind also. For that man, disappears the whole universe, as it were. This surging, moving, continuous struggle of forces stops for ever, and that which was manifesting itself as force and matter, as the struggles of nature, as nature itself, as heavens

and earths and plants and animals and men and
angels—all that becomes transfigured into one infinite,
unbreakable, unchangeable Existence; and the knowing man finds that he is one with that Existence. "Even
as clouds of various colours come before the sky,
remain there for a moment, and then vanish away,"
even so before this Soul come all these visions—of earth
and heaven, of the moon and the gods, of pleasures
and pains; but they all pass away, leaving behind
the infinite, unchangeable Spirit. The sky never
changes; it is the clouds that change. It is a mistake
to think that the Spirit changes. It is a mistake to
think that we are impure, that we are limited, that
we are separate. The real man is the one Existence.

Two questions now arise. The first is: "Can one
ever realize this truth? So far it is doctrine, philosophy;
but is it possible to realize it?" It is. There are men
still living for whom delusion has vanished for ever.
The second is: "Do they immediately die after such
realization?" Not so soon as we should think. Two
wheels joined by one pole are running together. If,
with an axe, I cut the pole asunder and get hold of
one of the wheels, it stops. But in the other wheel is
its past momentum; so it runs on a little and then falls
down. This pure and perfect Being, the Soul, is
one wheel, and this external hallucination of body and
mind is the other wheel, and they are joined together
by the pole of work, of karma. Knowledge is the axe
which will sever the bond between the two, and the
wheel of the Soul will stop—stop thinking that It is
coming and going, living and dying, stop thinking
that It is a part of nature and has wants and desires—

and will find that It is perfect, desireless. But in the other wheel, that of the body and mind, will be the momentum of past acts. So it will live for some time, until that momentum of past work is exhausted, until that momentum is worked out. Then the body and mind will fall, and the Soul be free. No more is there any going to heaven and coming back, not even any going to Brahmaloka or to any of the higher spheres; for where is the Soul to come from or to go to?

The man who has in this life attained to this state, for whom, for a minute at least, the ordinary vision of the world has changed and the reality has been apparent—he is called "free while living." This is the goal of the Vedāntist, to attain freedom in life.

Once in Western India I was travelling in the desert country. For days and days I travelled on foot through the desert; but to my surprise I saw every day beautiful lakes, with trees all round them, and the reflections of the trees upside down and vibrating there. "How wonderful it looks—and they call this a desert country!" I said to myself. Nearly a month I travelled, seeing these wonderful lakes and trees and plants. One day I was very thirsty and wanted to have a drink of water, so I started to go to one of these clear, beautiful lakes. But as I approached, it vanished; and with a flash the idea came to me, "This is the mirage, about which I have read all my life." And with that came also the idea that throughout the whole of that month, every day, I had been seeing the mirage and did not know it. The next morning I began my march. There was the lake again, but with it came also the idea that it was a mirage and not a true lake.

So is it with this universe. We are all travelling in this mirage of the world, day after day, month after month, year after year, not knowing that it is a mirage. One day it will disappear; but it will come back again. The body has to remain under the power of past karma, and so the mirage will come back. This world will come back to us so long as we are bound by karma: men, women, animals, plants, our attachments and duties, all will come back to us. But not with the same power; under the influence of the new knowledge the strength of karma will be broken, its poison will be lost. It will become transformed, for along with it will come the idea that we understand it now, that the sharp distinction between the reality and the mirage has been known. This world will not then be the same world as before.

There is, however, a danger here. We often see people taking up this philosophy and saying, "I am beyond all virtue and vice; so I am not bound by any moral laws; I may do anything I like." You can find many fools in this country at the present time saying, "I am not bound; I am God Himself; let me do anything I like." This is not right, although it is true that the Soul is beyond all laws, physical, mental, or moral. Within law is bondage; beyond law is freedom. It is also true that freedom is the nature of the Soul; it is Its birthright. That real freedom of the Soul shines through the veils of matter in the form of the apparent freedom of man. Every moment of your life you feel that you are free. We cannot live, talk, or breathe for a moment without feeling that we are free. But at the same time, a little thought shows us that we are like machines and not free. What is true, then? Is this idea of freedom a delusion? One party holds that the idea of freedom is a delusion; another says that the idea of bondage is a delusion. How does this happen?

Man is really free; the real man cannot but be free. It is when he comes into the world of māyā, into name and form, that he becomes bound. Free will is a misnomer. The will can never be free. How can it be? It is only when the real man has become bound that his will comes into existence, and not before. The will of man is bound, but that which is the foundation of that will is eternally free. So even in the state of bondage which we call human life or god-life, on earth or in heaven, there yet remains to us that recollection of the freedom which is ours by divine right. And consciously or unconsciously we are all struggling towards it.

When a man has attained his inner freedom, how can he be bound by any law? No law in this universe can bind him; for this universe itself is his. He is the whole universe. Either say he is the whole universe or say that to him there is no universe. How, then, can he have all these little ideas about sex and about country? How can he say, "I am a man," "I am a woman," "I am a child"? Are these not fantasies? He knows they are. How can he say that these are man's rights and these others are woman's rights? Nobody has rights; nobody exists separately. There is neither man nor woman; the Soul is sexless, eternally pure. It is a lie to say that I am a man or a woman or to say that I belong to this country or that. All the world is my country, the whole universe is mine, because I have clothed myself with it as my body.

Yet we see that there are people in this world who proclaim these doctrines and at the same time go on doing things which we should call filthy. And if we ask them why they do so, they tell us that we are deluded and that they can do nothing wrong. What is the test by which they are to be judged? The test is here. Though evil and good are both conditioned manifestations of the Soul, yet evil is the more external coating, and good is the inner coating of the Real Man, the Self. Unless a man cuts through the layer of evil he cannot reach the layer of good, and unless he has passed through both the layers, of good and of evil, he cannot reach the Self. He who reaches the Self—what remains attached to him? A little karma, a little bit of the momentum of his past life; but it is all good momentum. Until the bad momentum is entirely worked out and the past impurities are entirely burnt up, it is impossible for any man to see and realize Truth.

So what is left attached to the man who has reached the Self and seen Truth is the remnant of the good impressions of his past life, the good momentum. Even if he lives in the body and works incessantly, he works only to do good; his lips speak only benediction to all; his hands do only good works; his mind can think only good thoughts; his presence is a blessing wherever he goes. He is himself a living blessing. Such a man will, by his very presence, change even the most wicked persons into saints. Even if he does not speak, his very presence will be a blessing to mankind. Can such men do any evil? Can they do wicked deeds?

There is, you must remember, all the difference of pole from pole between realization and mere talking. Any fool can talk. Even parrots talk. Talking is one thing, and realizing is another. Philosophies and doctrines and arguments and books and theories and churches and sects and all such things are good as far as they go; but when realization comes these things drop away. For instance, maps are good, but when you see the country itself and look again at the maps, what a great difference you find! So those who have realized Truth do not require the ratiocinations of logic or any other gymnastics of the intellect to make them understand Truth; it is to them the life of their lives, concretized, made more than tangible. It is, as the sages of the Vedānta say, "even as a fruit in your hand": you can stand up and say, "It is here." So those who have realized Truth will stand up and say, "Here is the Self." You may argue with them by the year, but they will smile at you; they will regard it all as a child's prattle; they will let the child prattle on. They have realized Truth and are satisfied. Suppose you have seen a country, and a man comes and tries to argue with you that that country never existed. He may go on arguing indefinitely, but your only attitude of mind towards him will be to hold that the man is fit for a lunatic asylum. So the man of realization says, "All this talk in the world about its little religions is but prattle; realization is the soul, the very essence, of religion." Religion can be realized. Are you ready? Do you want it? You will get the realization if you do,

and then you will be truly religious. Until you have
attained realization there is no difference between
you and the atheists. The atheists are sincere, but
the man who says that he believes in religion and
never attempts to realize it is not sincere.

The next question is to know what comes after
realization. Suppose we have realized this oneness of
the universe, suppose we know that we are that one
Infinite Being; and suppose we have realized that
this Self is the only Existence, and that it is the same
Self which is manifested in all these various phenomenal forms—what becomes of us after that? Shall we
become inactive, get into a corner and sit down there
and die? "What good will it do to the world?"—that
old question! In the first place why should it do good
to the world? Is there any reason that it should? What
right has anyone to ask the question, "What good
will it do to the world?" What is meant by that? A
baby likes candies. Suppose you are conducting in-
vestigations in connexion with some aspect of electricity
and a baby asks you, "Does it buy candies?" "No,"
you answer. "Then what good will it do?" says the
baby. So men stand up and say: "What good will this
do to the world? Will it give us money?" "No." "Then
what good is there in it?" That is what men mean
by doing good to the world.

Yet religious realization does the greatest good to the
world. People are afraid that when they attain to it,
when they realize that there is but One, the foun-
tains of love will be dried up, everything in life will
go away, and all that they love will vanish for them,
as it were, in this life and in the life to come. People

never stop to think that the greatest workers in the world have been those who bestowed the least thought on their own individualities. Then alone does a man love when he finds that the object of his love is not any low, little, mortal thing. Then alone does a man love when he finds that the object of his love is not a clod of earth, but is the veritable God Himself. The wife will love the husband the more when she thinks that the husband is God Himself. The husband will love the wife the more when he knows that the wife is God Himself. That mother will love her children more who thinks that the children are God Himself. That man will love his greatest enemy who knows that that very enemy is God Himself. That man will love a holy man who knows that the holy man is God Himself, and that very man will also love the unholiest of men because he knows that the background of that unholiest of men is even He, the Lord. Such a man becomes a world-mover. For him the little self is dead and God stands in its place; for him the whole universe becomes transfigured. That which is painful and miserable will all vanish; struggles will all depart. Instead of being a prison-house, where every day we struggle and fight and compete for a morsel of bread, this universe will then be to us a playground. Beautiful will be this universe then! Such a man alone has the right to stand up and say, "How beautiful is this world!" He alone has the right to say that it is all good.

This will be the great good to the world resulting from such realization: If all mankind today realizes only a bit of that great truth, the aspect of the whole world will be changed; in place of fighting and

quarrelling there will be a reign of peace. This
indecent and brutal hurry which forces us to go
ahead of everyone else will then vanish from the
world. With it will vanish all fighting, with it will
vanish all hate, with it will vanish all jealousy; all
evil will vanish away for ever. Gods will live then
upon this earth. This very earth will become heaven
—and what evil can there be when gods are playing
with gods, when gods are working with gods, and
gods are loving gods? That is the great utility of divine
realization. Everything that you see in society will be
changed and transfigured then. No more will you think
of man as evil; and that is the first great gain. No
more will you stand up and sneeringly cast a glance
at a poor man or woman who has made a mistake. No
more, ladies, will you look down with contempt upon
the poor woman who walks the street in the night,
because you will see even there God Himself. No
more will you think of jealousy and punishments.
They will all vanish; and love, the great ideal of love,
will be so powerful that no whip and cord will be
necessary to guide mankind aright.

   If one millionth part of the men and women who
live in this world simply sit down and for a few
minutes say: "You are all God, O ye men and O ye
animals and living beings! You are all the manifestations of the one living Deity!" the whole world will be
changed in half an hour. Instead of throwing tremendous bomb-shells of hatred into every corner,
instead of projecting currents of jealousy and of evil
thought, in every country people will think that it
is all He. He is all that you see and feel. How can

you see evil unless there is evil in you? How can you see the thief unless he is there, sitting in your heart of hearts? How can you see the murderer unless you are yourself a murderer? Be good, and evil will vanish for you. The whole universe will thus be changed. This is the great gain to society. This is the great gain to humanity.

These thoughts were thought out, worked out, amongst individuals in ancient times in India. For various reasons, such as the exclusiveness of the teachers and foreign conquest, those thoughts were not allowed to spread. Yet they are grand truths, and wherever they have been working man has become divine. My whole life has been changed by the touch of one of these divine men, about whom I am going to speak to you next Sunday. The time is coming when these thoughts will be cast abroad over the whole world. Instead of living in monasteries, instead of being confined to books of philosophy to be studied only by the learned, instead of being the exclusive possession of sects and of a few of the learned, they will all be sown broadcast over the whole world, so that they may become the common property of the saint and the sinner, of men and women and children, of the learned and of the ignorant. They will then permeate the atmosphere of the world, and the very air that we breathe will say with every one of its vibrations, "Thou art That." And the whole universe, with its myriads of suns and moons, through everything that speaks, with one voice will say, "Thou art That."

PRACTICAL VEDĀNTA

PART I

(Delivered in London, November 10, 1896)

I HAVE BEEN ASKED to say something about the practical position of the Vedānta philosophy. As I have told you, theory is very good indeed; but how are we to carry it into practice? If it is absolutely impracticable, no theory is of any value whatever, except as intellectual gymnastics. Vedānta therefore, as a religion, must be intensely practical. We must be able to carry it out in every part of our lives. And not only this. The fictitious differentiation between religion and the life of the world must vanish; for Vedānta teaches Oneness—one life throughout. The ideals of religion must cover the whole field of life; they must enter into all our thoughts, and more and more into practice. I shall gradually take up the practical side as we proceed. But this series of lectures is intended to be a basis, and so we must first apply ourselves to theories and understand how they can be worked out, not only in forest caves but also in busy cities. And one peculiar feature we shall find is that many of these thoughts, instead of being the outcome of retirement into the forest, have emanated from persons whom we expect to lead the busiest lives—from ruling monarchs.

Śvetaketu was the son of Āruni, a sage, most probably a recluse. He was brought up in the forest,

208

but he went to the city of the Pānchālas and appeared at the court of King Pravāhana Jaivali. The king asked him, "Do you know how beings depart hence at death?" "No, sir." "Do you know how they return hither?" "No, sir." "Do you know the Way of the Fathers and the Way of the Gods?" "No, sir." Then the king asked other questions. Śvetaketu could not answer them. So the king told him that he knew nothing. The boy went back to his father and the father admitted that he himself could not answer these questions. It was not that he was unwilling to answer these questions; it was not that he was unwilling to teach the boy. But he did not know these things. So Śvetaketu returned to the king with his father and they both asked to be taught these secrets. The king said that these things had hitherto been known only among kings; the priests never knew them. He proceeded, however, to teach them what they desired to know.

In various Upanishads we find that this Vedānta philosophy is not the outcome of meditation in the forest only, but the very best parts of it were thought out and expressed by those brains which were busiest in the everyday affairs of life. We cannot conceive of any man busier than an absolute monarch, a man who rules over millions of people; and yet some of these rulers were deep thinkers. Everything goes to show that this philosophy is very practical. Later on, when we come to the Bhagavad Gītā—most of you, perhaps, have read it; it is the best commentary we have on the Vedānta philosophy—curiously enough the scene is laid on a battlefield, where Krishna teaches this philosophy to Arjuna. And the doctrine which stands out luminously on every page of the Gītā is that of intense activity, but in the midst of it, eternal calmness.

This is the secret of work, to attain which is the goal of Vedānta. Inactivity as we understand it, in the sense of passivity, certainly cannot be the goal. Were it so, then the walls around us would be the wisest of things; for they are inactive. Clods of earth, stumps of trees, would be the greatest sages in the world; for they are inactive. Nor does inactivity become activity when it is combined with passion. Real activity, which is the goal of Vedānta, is that which is combined with eternal calmness, the calmness which cannot be ruffled, the balance of mind which is not disturbed, no matter what happens. And we all know from experience that that is the best attitude for work.

I have been told many times that we cannot work if we do not have the passion which men generally feel for work. I also thought in that way years ago, but as I am growing older, getting more experience, I find it is not true. The less passion there is, the better we work. The calmer we are, the better it is for us and the greater is the amount of work we can do. When we let loose our feelings we waste so much energy, shatter our nerves, disturb our minds, and accomplish very little work. The energy which ought to have gone into work is spent as mere feeling, which counts for nothing. It is only when the mind is very calm and collected that the whole of its energy is spent in doing good work. And if you read the lives of the great workers the world has produced, you will find that they were wonderfully calm men. Nothing, as it were, could throw them off their balance. That is why the man who becomes angry never does a great amount of work, and the man whom nothing can make angry accomplishes so much. The man who gives way to anger or hatred or any other passion cannot work; he only breaks himself to pieces and does nothing practical. It is the calm, forgiving, equable, well balanced mind that does the greatest amount of work.

Vedānta preaches the ideal, and the ideal, as we know, is always far ahead of the real, of the practical, as we may call it. There are two tendencies in human nature: one to reconcile the ideal with life and the other to elevate life to the ideal. It is a great thing to understand this; for we are often tempted by the former. I think that I can do a certain kind of work. Most of it, perhaps, is bad; most of it, perhaps, has a motive power of passion behind it—anger, or greed, or selfishness. Now, if any man comes to preach to me a certain ideal, the first step towards which is to give up selfishness, to give up self-enjoyment, I think that that is impractical. But when a man brings an ideal which can be reconciled with my selfishness, I am glad and at once jump at it. That is the ideal for me. As the word *orthodox* has been manipulated into various forms, so has the word *practical*. "My doxy is orthodoxy; your doxy is heterodoxy." So with practicality. What I think is practical is to me the only practicality in the world. If I am a shopkeeper, I think shopkeeping the only practical pursuit in the world. If I am a thief, I think stealing is the best means of being practical; others are not practical. You see how we all use this word *practical* for things that *we* like and can do. Therefore I ask you to understand that Vedānta, though it is intensely practical, is always so in the sense of the ideal. It does not preach an impossible ideal, however high it may be, and it is high enough for an ideal.

In one word, this ideal is that you are divine. "Thou art That." This is the essence of Vedānta. After all its ramifications and intellectual gymnastics, you know the human soul to be pure and omniscient; you see that such superstitions as birth and death are entire nonsense when spoken of in connexion with the soul. The soul was never born and will never die, and all these ideas that we are going to die and are afraid to die are mere superstitions. And all such ideas as that we can do this, or cannot do that, are superstitions. We can do everything. Vedānta teaches men to have faith in themselves first. As certain religions of the world say that a man who does not believe in a Personal God outside himself is an atheist, so Vedānta says that a man who does not believe in himself is an atheist. Not believing in the glory of our own soul is what Vedānta calls atheism.

To many this is, no doubt, a terrible ideal, and most of us think that this ideal can never be reached; but Vedānta insists that it can be realized by everyone. One may be either man or woman or child; one may belong to any race—nothing will stand as a bar to the realization of this ideal, because, as Vedānta shows, it is realized already, it is already there. All the powers in the universe are already ours. It is we who have put our hands before our eyes and cry that it is dark. Know that there is no darkness around you. Take your hands away and there is the light which was from the beginning. Darkness never existed; weakness never existed. We who are fools cry that we are weak; we who are fools cry that we are impure. Thus Vedānta insists not only that the ideal is practical, but that it has been so always, and that this ideal, this Reality, is our own nature. Everything else that you see is false, untrue. As soon as you say, "I am a little mortal being," you are saying something which is not true, you are giving the lie to yourselves, you are hypnotizing yourselves into something vile and weak and wretched. Vedānta recognizes no sin; it recognizes only error. And the greatest error, it says, is to think that you are weak, that you are a sinner, a miserable creature, and that you have no power and cannot do this or that. Every time you think in that way, you rivet, as it were, one more link in the chain that binds you down, you add one more layer of hypnotism upon your soul. Therefore whosoever thinks he is weak is wrong, whosoever thinks he is impure is wrong, and is throwing a bad thought into the world.

This we must always bear in mind: In Vedānta there is no attempt at reconciling the present life, the hypnotized life, this false life which we have assumed, with the ideal; but this false life must go, and the real life, which has always existed, must manifest itself, must shine out. No man becomes purer and purer; it is a matter of greater manifestation of the perfection that has always been in him. The veil drops away, and the native purity of the soul begins to manifest itself. Everything is ours already—infinite purity, freedom, love, and power.

Vedānta also says that this can be realized not only in the depths of forests or in caves, but by men in all possible conditions of life. We have seen that the people who discovered these truths were neither living in caves or forests nor following the ordinary vocations of life, but were men who, we have every reason to believe, led the busiest of lives, men who had to command armies, to sit on thrones and look to the welfare of millions—and all this in the days of absolute monarchy, and not in these days when a king is to a great extent a mere figurehead. Yet they could find time to think out all these thoughts, to realize them, and to teach them to humanity. How much more, then, should they be practical for us, whose lives, compared with theirs, are lives of leisure! That we cannot realize them is a shame to us, seeing that we are comparatively free all the time and have very little to do. My requirements are as nothing compared with those of an ancient absolute monarch. My wants are as nothing compared with the demands of Arjuna on the battlefield of Kurukshetra, commanding a huge army; and yet he could find time in the midst of the din and turmoil of battle to talk the highest philosophy and to carry it into his life. Surely we ought to be able to do as much in this life of ours, comparatively free, easy, and comfortable. Most of us here have more time than we think we have, if we really want to use it for good. With the amount of freedom we have, we can attain to two hundred ideals in this life, if we will. But we must not degrade the ideal to the actual. Here is a great danger. There are persons who teach us how to make special excuses for all our foolish wants and foolish desires; and we think that their ideal is the only ideal we need have. But it is not so. Vedānta teaches no such thing. The actual should be harmonized with the ideal; the present life should be made to coincide with life eternal.

For you must always remember that the central ideal of Vedānta is Oneness. There are no two in anything —no two lives or even two different kinds of life for the two worlds. You will find the Vedas speaking, at first, of heavens and things like that; but later on, when they come to the highest ideals of their philosophy, they brush away all these things. There is but one Life, one World, one Existence. Everything is that One; the differences are of degree and not of kind. The differences between our lives are not of kind. Vedānta entirely denies such ideas as that animals are essentially separate from men and that they were made and created by God to be used for our food.

Some people have been kind enough to start an anti-vivisection society. I asked a member, "Why do you think, my friend, that it is quite lawful to kill animals for food, and not to kill one or two for scientific experiments?" He replied, "Vivisection is most horrible, but animals have been given to us for food."

Oneness includes all animals. If man is immortal, so also are the animals. The differences are only of degree and not of kind. The amoeba and I are the same; the difference is only one of degree; and from the standpoint of the highest life, all differences vanish. A man may see a great deal of difference between grass and a little tree, but if he mounts very high, the grass and

the biggest tree will appear much the same. So, from
the standpoint of the highest ideal, the lowest animal
and the highest man are the same. If you believe there
is a God, then to Him the animals and the highest
creatures must be the same. A God who is partial to
His children called men, and cruel to His children
called brute beasts, is worse than a demon. I would
rather die a hundred times than worship such a God.
My whole life would be a fight with such a God. But
there is no difference from the standpoint of God; and
those who say that there is are irresponsible, heartless
people, who do not know.

Here, then, is a case of the word *practical* used in a
wrong sense. We eat meat not because animals have
been given to us for food, but because we want to. I
myself may not be a very strict vegetarian, but I
understand the ideal. When I eat meat I know it is
wrong. Even if I am bound to eat it under certain
circumstances, I know it is cruel. I must not drag my
ideal down to the actual and give excuses for my weak
conduct. The ideal is not to eat flesh, not to injure
any being; for all animals are my brothers. If you can
think of them as your brothers, you have made a little
headway towards the brotherhood of all souls, not to
speak of the brotherhood of man! But to carry this out
is no child's-play. You generally find that this is not
very acceptable to many, because it teaches them to
give up the actual and go towards the ideal. But if
you bring out a theory which can be reconciled with
their present conduct, they regard it as entirely practical.

There is a strongly conservative tendency in human

nature; we do not like to move one step forward. I think of mankind as being like those I have read about who have become frozen in the snow. All such, they say, want to go to sleep, and if you try to drag them out, they say: "Let me sleep. It is so beautiful to sleep in the snow"; and they die there in that sleep. So is our nature. That is what we are doing all our life—getting frozen from the feet upwards and yet wanting to sleep. Therefore you must struggle towards the ideal; and if a man comes who wants to bring that ideal down to your level and teach a religion which does not carry out that highest ideal, do not listen to him. To me that is an impracticable religion. But if a man teaches a religion which presents the highest ideal, I am ready for him.

Beware when anyone is trying to give excuses for sense vanities and sense weaknesses. If anyone wants to preach that way to us—poor, sense-bound clods of earth that we have made ourselves—by following that teaching we shall never progress. I have seen many of these things; I have had some experience of the world; and my country is the land where religious sects grow like mushrooms. Every year new sects arise. But one thing I have marked: that it is only those who never want to reconcile the man of flesh with the man of truth who make progress. Wherever there is this false idea of reconciling fleshly vanities with the highest ideals, of dragging down God to the level of man, there comes decay. Man should not be degraded to worldly slavery, but should be raised up to God.

At the same time, there is another side to the question. We must not look down with contempt on others.

All of us are going towards the same goal. The difference between weakness and strength is one of degree.
The difference between virtue and vice is one of degree. The difference between heaven and hell is one
of degree. The difference between life and death is
one of degree. All differences in this world are of
degree, and not of kind, because Oneness is the secret
of everything. All is the One, and the One manifests
Itself either as thought or life or soul or body. This
being so, we have no right to look down with contempt
upon those who are not developed exactly in the same
degree as we are. Condemn none. If you can stretch
out a helping hand, do so; if you cannot, fold your
hands, bless your brothers, and let them go their own
way. Dragging down and condemning is not the way
to work. Never is work accomplished in that way. We
spend our energies in condemning others. Criticism
and condemnation are a vain way of spending our
energies; for in the long run we come to learn that all
are seeking the same thing, are more or less approaching the same ideal, and that most of our differences
are merely differences of expression.

Take the idea of sin. I was telling you just now the
Vedāntic idea of it. The other view is that man is a
sinner. They are practically the same, only the one
takes the positive and the other the negative side. One
shows man his strength, and the other, his weakness.
There may be weakness, says Vedānta, but never mind,
we want to grow. Disease existed in man as soon as he
was born. Everyone knows his disease; it requires no
one to tell us what our diseases are. But thinking all
the time that we are diseased will not cure us. Medi-

cine is necessary. In our heart of hearts we all know our weaknesses. But, says Vedānta, being reminded of weakness does not help much. Give strength. And strength does not come by thinking of weakness all the time. The remedy for weakness is not brooding over weakness, but thinking of strength. Teach men of the strength that is already within them. Instead of telling them that they are sinners, Vedānta takes the opposite position and says, "You are pure and perfect, and what you call sin does not belong to you." Sins are very low degrees of Self-manifestation; manifest the Self in a high degree. That is the one thing to remember. All of us can do that. Never say no; never say, "I cannot"; for you are infinite. Even time and space are as nothing compared with your nature. You can do anything and everything; you are almighty.

These are the principles of ethics; but we shall now come down lower and work out the details. We shall see how Vedānta can be carried into our everyday life —the city life, the country life, the national life, and the home life of every nation. For if a religion cannot help a man wherever he may be, wherever he stands, it is not of much use; it will remain only a theory for the chosen few. A religion, to help mankind, must be ready and able to help a man in whatever condition he may be—in servitude or in freedom, in the depths of degradation or on the heights of purity. Everywhere, equally, it should be able to come to his aid. The ideal of Vedānta, the ideal of religion—or whatever you may prefer to call it—will be fulfilled only if it is capable of performing this great and noble function.

The ideal of faith in ourselves is of the greatest help

to us. If faith in ourselves had been more extensively
taught and practised, I am sure a very large portion of
the evils and miseries that we have would have vanished. Throughout the history of mankind, if any one
motive power has been more potent than others in the
lives of great men and women, it is that of faith in
themselves. Born with the consciousness that they
were to be great, they became great. Let a man go
down as low as possible, yet there must come a time
when out of sheer desperation he will take an upward
curve and learn to have faith in himself. But it is better
for us that we should know it from the very first. Why
should we have all these bitter experiences in order to
gain faith in ourselves? We can see that all the difference there is between man and man is due to the
existence or non-existence of faith in himself. Faith in
ourselves will do everything. I have experienced it in
my own life, and am still doing so, and as I grow older
that faith is becoming stronger and stronger. He is an
atheist who does not believe in himself. The old religions said that he who did not believe in God was
the atheist. The new religion says that he is the atheist
who does not believe in himself. But it is not selfish
faith, because Vedānta, again, is the doctrine of Oneness. It means faith in all because you are all. Love
for yourself means love for all—love for animals, love
for everything; for you are all. This is the great faith
which will make the world better. I am sure of that.

He is the highest man who can say with truth, "I
know all about myself." Do you know how much
energy, how many powers, how many forces, are still
lurking within that frame of yours? What scientist has

known all that is in man? Millions of years have passed since man first came here, and yet but one infinitesimal part of his powers has been manifested. Therefore you must not say that you are weak. How do you know what possibilities lie behind that degradation on the surface? You know but little of that which is within you. For behind you is the Ocean of infinite power and blessedness.

"This Ātman is first to be heard of." Hear day and night that you are that Soul. Repeat it to yourselves day and night till it enters into your very veins, till it tingles in every drop of blood, till it is in your flesh and bone. Let the whole body be full of that one idea: "I am the birthless, the deathless, the blissful, the omniscient, the omnipotent, ever glorious Soul." Think of it day and night; think of it till it becomes part and parcel of your life. Meditate upon it. And out of that will come work. "Out of the fullness of the heart the mouth speaketh," and out of the fullness of the heart the hand worketh also. Action will come. Fill yourselves with the ideal; remember it well before you take up any work. Then all your actions will be glorified, transformed, deified, by the very power of this thought. If matter is powerful, thought is omnipotent. Bring this thought to bear upon your life, fill yourselves with the thought of your almightiness, your majesty, and your glory.

Would to God no superstitions had been put into your head! Would to God we had not been surrounded from our birth by all these superstitious influences and paralysing ideas of our weakness and vileness! Would to God that mankind had had an easier path through which to attain to the noblest and highest truths! But man has to pass through all this; do not make the path more difficult for those who come after you.

These are sometimes terrible doctrines to teach. I know people who get frightened at these ideas; but for those who want to be practical, this is the first thing to learn. Never tell yourselves or others that you are weak. Do good if you can, but do not injure the world. You know in your inmost heart that many of your limited ideas—this humbling of yourself, and praying and weeping to imaginary beings—are superstitions. Tell me one case where these prayers have been answered from outside. All the answers came from your own hearts. You know there are no ghosts, but no sooner are you in the dark than you feel a little creepy sensation. That is because in your childhood you have had all these fearful ideas put into your heads. But do not teach these things to others—through fear of society and public opinion, or for fear of incurring the hatred of friends, or for fear of losing cherished superstitions. Be masters of all these. What is there to be taught in religion more than the oneness of the universe, and faith in oneself? All the efforts of mankind for thousands of years past have been directed towards this one goal, and mankind is yet to work it out. It is your turn now and you already know the truth. For it has been taught on all sides. Not only philosophy and psychology, but the materialistic sciences have declared it. Where is the scientific man today who fears to acknowledge the truth of this oneness of the universe?

Who is there who dares talk of many worlds? All these are superstitions.

There is only one Life, one World; and this one Life, this one World, appears to us to be manifold. This manifoldness is like a dream. When you dream, one dream passes away and another comes. None of your dreams are real. The dreams come one after another; scene after scene unfolds before you. So it is in this world of ninety per cent misery and ten per cent happiness. Perhaps after a while it will appear as ninety per cent happiness, and we shall call it heaven. But a time comes to the sage when the whole thing vanishes and this world appears as God Himself, and his own soul as that God. It is not true that there are many worlds; it is not true that there are many lives. All this manifoldness is the manifestation of that One. That One is manifesting Himself as many—as matter, spirit, mind, thought, and everything else. Therefore the first step for us to take is to teach the truth to ourselves and to others. Let the world resound with this ideal and let superstitions vanish. Tell it to men who are weak, and persist in telling it.

"You are the Pure One. Awake and arise, Almighty One! This sleep does not become you. Awake and arise; it does not befit you. Think not that you are weak and miserable. Almighty One, arise and awake, and manifest your true nature. It is not fitting that you think yourself a sinner. It is not fitting that you think yourself weak." Say that to the world, say it to yourselves, and see what a practical result follows; see how with an electric flash the truth is manifested, how everything is changed. Tell it to men and show them their power. Then they will learn how to apply it in their daily lives.

To be able to use what we call viveka, discrimination, to learn how, in every moment of our lives, in every one of our actions, to discriminate between right and wrong, true and false, we shall have to know the test of truth, which is purity, oneness. Everything that makes for oneness is truth. Love is truth and hatred is falsehood, because hatred makes for multiplicity. It is hatred that separates man from man; therefore it is wrong and false. It is a disintegrating power; it separates and destroys. Love unites; love makes for that oneness. You become one—the mother with the child, families with the city; human beings become one with the animals. For love is Existence, God Himself, and all this is the manifestation of that one Love, more or less expressed. The differences are only of degree; it is the manifestation of that one Love throughout. Therefore in all our actions we have to judge whether our act is making for diversity or for oneness. If it makes for diversity, we have to give it up, but if for oneness, we may be sure it is good. So with our thoughts; we have to decide whether they make for disintegration, multiplicity, or for oneness, binding soul to soul and thus generating a great force. If they do this, we will take them up, and if not, we will throw them off as wicked.

The whole idea of Vedāntic ethics is that it does not depend on anything unknowable, nor does it teach anything unknown. On the contrary, it teaches, in the language of St. Paul: "Whom therefore ye ignorantly worship, him declare I unto you." It is through the

Self that you know everything. I see this chair; but to see the chair, first I have to perceive myself and then the chair. It is in and through the Self that the chair is perceived. It is in and through the Self that you are known to me, that the whole world is known to me; and therefore to say that this Self is unknown is sheer nonsense. Take away the Self and the whole universe vanishes. In and through the Self all knowledge comes. Therefore It is the best known of all. It is yourself— that which you call "I." You may wonder how this "I" of me can be the "I" of you. You may wonder how this limited "I" can be the unlimited Infinite. But it is so. The limited "I" is a mere fiction. The Infinite has been covered up, as it were, and a little of It is being manifested as the "I." Limitation can never come upon the unlimited; it is a fiction. The Self is known, there- fore, to every one of us—man, woman, or child—and even to animals. Without knowing It we can neither live nor move nor have our being; without knowing this Lord of all we cannot breathe or live a second. The God of Vedānta is the most known of all and is not the outcome of imagination.

If this is not preaching a practical God—how else could you preach a practical God? Where is there a more practical God than Him whom I see before me, a God omnipresent, in every being, more real than anything we see through our senses? For you are He, the omnipresent God Almighty, and if I say you are not, I tell an untruth. I know it, whether at all times I realize it or not. He is the Oneness, the Unity of all, the Reality of all life and all existence.

These ideas of the ethics of Vedānta have to be

worked out in detail, and therefore you must have patience. As I have told you, we want to take the subject in detail and work it out thoroughly to see how these ideas have grown from a very low level and how the one great idea of oneness has developed and become shaped into the Universal Love. We ought to study all these in order to avoid dangers.

The world cannot find time to work it out from the lowest steps. But what is the use of our standing on higher steps if we cannot give the truth to others coming afterwards? Therefore it is better to study it in all its workings; and first it is absolutely necessary to clear the intellectual portion, although we know that intellectuality is almost nothing; for it is the heart that is of most importance. It is through the heart that the Lord is seen, and not through the intellect. The intellect is a street-cleaner, cleansing the path for us, a secondary worker, a policeman. But the policeman is not a positive necessity for the workings of society; he is only to stop disturbances, to check wrong-doing. And that is all the work required of the intellect. When you read intellectual books, you feel when you have mastered them, "Bless the Lord that I am out of them!" because the intellect is blind and cannot move of itself; it has neither hands nor feet. It is feeling that works, that moves with speed infinitely superior to that of electricity or anything else. Do you feel?—that is the question. If you do, you will see the Lord. The feeling that you have today will be intensified, deified, raised to the highest level, till you feel the oneness in everything, till you feel God in yourself and in others. The intellect can never do that. "Different methods of speaking words, different methods of explaining the texts of books—these are for the enjoyment of the learned, not for the salvation of the soul."

Those of you who have read Thomas à Kempis know how on every page he insists on this, and almost every holy man in the world has insisted on it. Intellect is necessary; for without it we fall into crude errors and make all sorts of mistakes. Intellect checks these. But beyond that do not try to build anything upon it. It is an inactive, secondary help; the real help is feeling, love. Do you feel for others? If you do, you are growing in oneness. If you do not feel for others, you may be the greatest intellectual giant ever born, but you will be nothing; you are but dry intellect and you will remain so. And if you feel, even if you cannot read any book and do not know any language, you are on the right way. The Lord is yours.

Do you not know, from the history of the world, where the power of the prophets lay? Where was it? In the intellect? Did any of them write a fine book on philosophy, on the most intricate ratiocinations of logic? Not one of them. They only spoke a few words. Feel like Christ and you will be a Christ; feel like Buddha and you will be a Buddha. It is feeling that is the life, the strength, the vitality, without which no amount of intellectual activity can reach God. Intellect is like limbs without the power of locomotion. It is only when feeling enters and gives the intellect motion that it moves and works on others. That is so all over the world, and it is a thing which you must always remember. It is one of the most practical things in Vedāntic morality; for it is the teaching of Vedānta that you are all prophets and that you all must be prophets.

Scripture is not the proof of your conduct, but you are the proof of scripture. How do you know that a book teaches truth? Because you are truth and feel it. That is what Vedānta says. What is the proof of the Christs and Buddhas of the world? That you and I feel like them. That is how you and I understand that they were true. Our prophet soul is the proof of their prophet soul. Your godhead is the proof of God Himself. If you are not a prophet there never has been anything true of God. If you are not God there never was any God and never will be.

This, says Vedānta, is the ideal to follow. Every one of us will have to become a prophet. You are that already; only *know* it. Never think there is anything impossible for the soul. It is the greatest heresy to think so. If there is sin, this is the only sin: to say that you are weak or others are weak.

PRACTICAL VEDĀNTA

PART II

(Delivered in London, November 12, 1896)

I WILL RELATE TO YOU a very ancient story from the *Chhāndogya Upanishad*, which tells how knowledge came to a boy. The story itself is crude, but we shall find that it contains a principle.

A young boy said to his mother: "I am going to study the Vedas. Tell me the name of my father and my caste." The mother was not a married woman, and in India the child of a woman who has not been married is considered an outcaste; he is not recognized by society and is not entitled to study the Vedas. So the poor mother said: "My child, I do not know your family name. I used to serve different people. You were born when I was in service. I do not know who your father is. But my name is Jabālā and your name is Satyakāma."

The boy went to a sage and asked to be taken as a student. The sage asked him, "What is the name of your father, and what is your caste?" The boy repeated to him what he had heard from his mother. The sage at once said: "None but a brāhmin could speak such a damaging truth about himself. You are a brāhmin and I will teach you. You have not swerved from truth." So he kept the boy with him and educated him.

229

Now we come to some of the peculiar methods of
education in ancient India. This teacher gave Satyakāma four hundred lean, weak cows to take care of
and sent him to the forest. There he went and lived
for some time. The teacher had told him to come back
when the herd had increased to one thousand. After
a few years, one day Satyakāma heard a big bull in
the herd saying to him: "We are a thousand now;
take us back to your teacher. I will teach you a little
of Brahman." "Go on, sir," said Satyakāma. Then the
bull said: "The East is a part of the Lord; so is the
West; so is the South; so is the North. The four cardinal points are the four parts of Brahman. Fire will
also teach you something of Brahman."

In those days fire was worshipped as a special symbol of Brahman, and every student had to light the
sacrificial fire and make offerings. So on the following
day Satyakāma started for his guru's house, and when
in the evening he had offered his oblation and worshipped the fire, and was sitting near it, he heard a
voice come from the fire: "O Satyakāma!" "Speak,
Lord," said Satyakāma. (Perhaps you remember a very
similar story in the Old Testament: how Samuel heard
a mysterious voice.) The fire said: "O Satyakāma, I
will teach you a little of Brahman. This earth is a
portion of that Brahman. The sky and heaven are
portions of It. The ocean is a part of that Brahman."
Then the fire said that a certain bird would also teach
him something.

Satyakāma continued his journey, and on the next
day, when he had performed his evening sacrifice, a
swan came to him and said: "I will teach you some-

thing about Brahman. This fire which you worship, O Satyakāma, is a part of that Brahman. The sun is a part, the moon is a part, lightning is a part of that Brahman. A bird called Madgu will tell you more about It." The next evening that bird came, and a similar voice was heard by Satyakāma: "I will tell you something about Brahman. Breath is a part of Brahman, sight is a part, hearing is a part, the mind is a part."

Then the boy arrived at his teacher's place and presented himself before him with due reverence. No sooner had the teacher seen him than he said: "Satyakāma, your face shines like the face of a knower of Brahman! Who, then, has taught you?" "Creatures other than men," replied Satyakāma. "But I wish that you should teach me, sir. For I have heard from men like you that knowledge learnt from a guru alone leads to the supreme good." Then the sage taught him the same knowledge that he had received from the others. "And nothing was left out, yea, nothing was left out."

Now, apart from the allegories in what the bull, the fire, and the birds taught, we see the tendency of the thought and the direction in which it was going in those days. The great idea of which we here see the germ is that all these voices are inside ourselves. As we understand these truths better, we find that the voice is in our own heart. The student understood that all the time he was hearing the truth; but his explanation was not correct. He was interpreting the voice as coming from the external world, while all the time it was within him.

The second idea that we get is that of making the

knowledge of Brahman practical. The world is always
seeking the practical possibilities of religion, and we
find in these stories how it was becoming more and
more practical every day. The truth was shown through
everything with which the students were familiar.
The fire they were worshipping was Brahman, the
earth was a part of Brahman, and so on.

The next story refers to Upakośala Kamalāyana, a
disciple of this Satyakāma, who wanted to be taught
by him and dwelt with him for some time. Now,
Satyakāma went away on a journey, and the student
became very downhearted; and when the teacher's
wife came and asked him why he was not eating, the
boy said, "I am too unhappy to eat." Then a voice
came from the fire he was worshipping, and said: "Life
is Brahman; Brahman is ākāśa; Brahman is happiness.
Know Brahman." "I know, sir," the boy replied, "that
life is Brahman, but that It is ākāśa and happiness I
do not know." Then the voice explained that the two
words ākāśa and happiness signified one thing in reality, that is, Pure Intelligence, which resides in the
heart. So it taught him that Brahman is life and the
ākāśa in the heart. Next the fire taught: "This earth,
food, fire, and the sun, which you worship, are forms
of Brahman. The Person who is seen in the sun—I
am He. He who knows this and meditates on Him—
all his sins vanish and he has long life and becomes
happy. He who lives in the cardinal points, the moon,
the stars, and water—I am He. He who lives in this
life, the ākāśa, the heavens, and lightning—I am He."

Here too we see the same idea of practical religion.
The things which they were worshipping, such as

fire, the sun, the moon, and so forth, and with which they were familiar, form the subject of the stories, which explain them and give them a higher meaning. And this is the real, practical side of Vedānta. It does not destroy the world, but it explains it; it does not destroy the person, but it explains him; it does not destroy the individuality, but it explains it by showing the real individuality. It does not show that this world is vain and does not exist, but it says, "Understand what this world is, so that it may not hurt you."

The voice did not say to Satyakāma that the fire which he was worshipping, or the sun, or the moon, or the lightning, or anything else, was all wrong; but it showed him that the same Spirit which was inside the sun and moon and lightning and fire and the earth was in him, so that everything became transformed, as it were, in the eyes of Satyakāma. The fire, which before had been merely a material fire in which to make oblations, assumed a new aspect and became God. The earth became transformed, life became transformed, the sun, the moon, the stars, lightning, everything became transformed and deified. Their real nature was known. The theme of Vedānta is to see the Lord in everything, to see things in their real nature, not as they appear to be.

Then another lesson is taught in the Upanishads: "He who shines through the eyes is Brahman. He is the Beautiful One. He is the Shining One. He shines in all these worlds." A certain peculiar light, a commentator says, which radiates from the eyes of the pure man, is what is meant by the light in the eyes; and it is said that when a man is pure such a light will

shine in his eyes, and that light belongs really to the
Soul within, which is everywhere. It is the same light
that shines in the planets, in the stars, and in the sun.

I will now read to you some other doctrines of these
ancient Upanishads, about birth and death and so on.
Perhaps they will interest you. Śvetaketu went to the
king of the Pānchālas, and the king asked him: "Do
you know where people go when they die? Do you
know how they come back? Do you know why the
earth is neither full nor empty?" The boy replied that
he did not know. Then he went to his father and
asked him the same questions. The father said, "I do
not know," and they both returned to the king. The
king said that this knowledge was never known to the
priests; it was known only to the kings, and that was
why kings ruled the world. They both served the king
for some time, and at last the king said he would teach
them. "The other world, O Gautama, is the fire. The
sun is its fuel, the rays are the smoke, the day is the
flame, the moon is the embers, and the stars are the
sparks. In this fire the gods pour the libation of faith,
and from this libation King Soma is born." So on he
goes. The gist of the teaching is this: "You need not
make oblation in that little fire; the whole world is the
fire, and this oblation, this worship, is continually
going on. The gods and the angels and everybody are
worshipping it. Man is the greatest symbol of fire—
the body of man."

Here also we see the ideal becoming practical.
Brahman is seen in everything. The principle that
underlies all these stories is that invented symbolism
may be good and helpful, but symbols better than

any we can invent already exist. You may invent an image through which to worship God, but a better image already exists—the living man. You may build a temple in which to worship God, and that may be good, but a better one, a much higher one, already exists—the human body.

You remember that the Vedas have two parts: the ceremonial and the philosophical. In time, ceremonies had multiplied and become so intricate that it was almost hopeless to disentangle them; and so in the Upanishads the ceremonies are almost discarded, but gently, by having their deeper meaning explained. We see that in olden times people had had these oblations and sacrifices. Then the philosophers came, and instead of snatching away the symbols from the hands of the ignorant, instead of taking the negative position which we unfortunately find so general among modern reformers, they gave them something in their place. "Here is the symbol of fire," they said. "Very good. But here is another symbol of fire—the earth, where sacrifice is going on day and night. What a grand symbol! Here is this little temple. But the whole universe is a temple; a man can worship anywhere. There are altars made by men; but here is the greatest of altars, the living, conscious human body; and worship at this altar is far higher than the worship of any dead symbols."

We now come to a peculiar doctrine. I do not understand much of it myself. I shall describe it to you and see if you can make something out of it. When a man who has by meditation purified himself and got knowledge dies, he first goes to light, then from light

to day, from day to the bright half of the moon, from
there to the six months when the sun goes to the
north, from there to the year, from the year to the
sun, from the sun to the moon, from the moon to
lightning, and when he comes to the sphere of lightning he meets a person who is not human, and that
person leads him to the conditioned Brahman. This is
the Way of the Gods. When sages and wise persons
die they go that way and they do not return. What
is meant by this month and year and all these things,
no one understands clearly. Each one gives his own
meaning, and some say it is all nonsense. What is
meant by going to the world of the moon and of the
sun, and by this person who comes to help the soul
after it has reached the sphere of lightning, no one
knows.

There is an idea among the Hindus that the moon
is a place where life exists, and we shall see how life
has come from there. When those who have not attained to knowledge, but have done good work in this
life, die, they first go through smoke, then to night,
then to the dark half of the moon, then to the six
months when the sun goes to the south, and from
there to the region of their forefathers, then to the
ākāśa, then to the region of the moon, and there become the food of the gods, and later are born as gods
and live there so long as their good works permit. This
is called the Way of the Fathers. And when the effect
of the good works is finished they come back to earth
by the same route. They first become ākāśa, and then
air, and then smoke, and then mist, and then cloud,
and then they fall upon the earth as raindrops; then

they get into food, which is eaten by human beings, and finally become their children. Those whose works have been very good are born in good families, and those whose works have been bad are born in bad families, and even in animal bodies. Again, those who do not travel either by the Way of the Gods or by the Way of the Fathers—those who have done vile deeds —become insects, being born and dying almost instantly. That is why the earth is neither full nor empty.

We can get several ideas from this also, and later on perhaps we shall be able to understand it better and speculate a little upon what it means. The last part, which deals with how those who have been in heaven return, is clearer perhaps than the first part; but the whole idea seems to be that there is no true immortality without realizing God. Some people who have not realized God, but have done good work in this world with a view to enjoying the results, go, when they die, through this and that place until they reach heaven, and there they are born in the same way as we are here, as children of the gods, and they live there so long as their good works permit. Out of this comes one basic idea of Vedānta, namely, that everything which has name and form is transient. This earth is transient, because it has name and form, and so the heavens must be transient, because there also name and form remain. A heaven which was eternal would be a contradiction in terms, because everything that has name and form must begin in time, exist in time, and end in time. These are settled doctrines of Vedānta. And therefore the heavens are given up.

We have seen that in the Samhitās the idea of

heaven was that it was eternal—much the same idea
as is prevalent among Mohammedans and Christians.
The Mohammedans concretize it a little more. They
say that it is a place where there are gardens, beneath
which rivers run. In the desert of Arabia water is very
desirable; so the Mohammedan always conceives his
heaven as containing much water. I was born in a
country where there are six months of rain every year.
I should think of heaven, I suppose, as a dry place,
and so also would the English people. These heavens
in the Samhitās are eternal, and the departed have
beautiful bodies and live with their forefathers and
are happy ever afterwards. There they meet with their
parents, children, and other relatives, and lead very
much the same sort of life as here, only much happier.
All the difficulties and obstructions to happiness in this
life have vanished, and only its good parts and enjoyments remain.

But however comfortable mankind may consider
this state of things, truth is one thing and comfort is
another. There are cases where truth is not comfortable until we reach its climax. Human nature is very
conservative. It does something, and having once done
that, finds it hard to get out of it. The mind will not
receive new thoughts, because they bring discomfort.

In the Upanishads we see that a tremendous de-
parture is made. It is declared that these heavens in
which men live with their ancestors after death cannot
be permanent, seeing that everything which has name
and form must die. If there are heavens with form,
these heavens must vanish in the course of time; they
may last millions of years, but there will come a time

when they must go. With this idea comes another: that these souls must come back to earth—that heavens are places where they enjoy the results of their good works, and after these results are exhausted they must come back to this earth-life again.

One thing is clear from this: that mankind had a perception of the philosophy of causation even at that early time. Later on we shall see how our philosophers bring this out in the language of philosophy and logic; but here it is almost in the language of children.

You may remark one thing in reading these books: that it is all internal perception. If you ask me if all this can be practical, my answer is, it was practical first and philosophical next. You can see that these things first were perceived and realized, and then written down. This earth spoke to the early thinkers. Birds spoke to them, animals spoke to them; the sun and moon spoke to them, and little by little they understood things and got into the heart of nature. Not by cogitation, not by the force of logic, not by picking the brains of others and writing a big book, as is the fashion in modern times, not even as I do, by taking up one of their writings and making a long lecture, but by patient investigation and discovery, they found out the truth. Their essential method was practice, and so it must be always. Religion is ever a practical science, and there never was or will be any theoretical religion. It is practice first, and knowledge afterwards.

The idea that souls come back is already there. Those persons who do good work with the idea of a result get the result, but it is not permanent. There we have the idea of causation very beautifully put forward.

The effect is only commensurate with the cause. As the cause is, so the effect will be. The cause being finite, the effect must be finite. If the cause is eternal the effect will be eternal; but all these causes—doing good work and all other things—are only finite causes, and as such cannot produce an infinite result.

We now come to the other side of the question. Just as there cannot be an eternal heaven, so, on the same grounds, there cannot be an eternal hell. Suppose I am a very wicked man, doing evil every minute of my life. Still, my whole life here, compared with my eternal life, is nothing. If there were an eternal punishment, it would mean that there was an infinite effect produced by a finite cause, which cannot be. If I do good all my life I cannot have an eternal heaven; it would be making the same mistake.

We have already spoken of the Way of the Gods and the Way of the Fathers. But there is a third course, which applies to those who have known Truth, to those who have realized It. This is the only way to get beyond the veil of māyā—to realize what Truth is. And the Upanishads indicate what is meant by realizing Truth. It means recognizing neither good nor bad, but knowing that all comes from the Self, and that the Self is in everything. It means denying the universe, shutting your eyes to it, seeing the Lord in hell as well as in heaven, seeing the Lord in death as well as in life. This is the line of thought in the passage I have read to you. The earth is a symbol of the Lord, the sky is the Lord—everything is Brahman. And this is to be seen, realized, not simply talked or thought about. We can see as its logical consequence that when the soul has realized that everything is full of the Lord, of Brahman, it will not care whether it goes to heaven or hell or anywhere else, whether it is born again on this earth or in heaven. These things have ceased to have any meaning for that soul, because every place is the same, every place is the temple of the Lord, every place has become holy, and the presence of the Lord is all that it sees in heaven or hell or anywhere else. Neither good nor bad, neither life nor death—only the one infinite Brahman exists.

According to Vedānta, when a man has arrived at that perception he has become free, and he is the only man who is fit to live in this world. Others are not. The man who sees evil—how can he live in this world? His life is a mass of misery. The man who sees dangers —his life is a misery. The man who sees death—his life is a misery. That man alone can live in this world, he alone can say, "I enjoy this life and I am happy in this life," who has seen Truth. And Truth exists in everything.

By the bye, I may tell you that the idea of hell does not occur anywhere in the Vedas. It comes with the Purānas, much later. The worst punishment, according to the Vedas, is coming back to earth, having another life in this world. From the very first we see that the thought is taking an impersonal turn. The ideas of punishment and reward are very material, and they are consonant only with the idea of a Personal God who loves one and hates another just as we do. Punishment and reward are admissible only with the existence of such a God. They had such a God in the Samhitās, and there we find the idea of fear entering;

but as soon as we come to the Upanishads, the idea of
fear vanishes and the idea of the Impersonal takes
its place.

It is naturally the hardest thing for man to understand, this idea of the Impersonal, for he is always
clinging to the Personal. Even people who are considered great thinkers get disgusted at the idea of the
Impersonal God. But to me it seems absurd to think
of God as if He were an embodied man. Which is the
higher idea, a living God or a dead God? A God whom
nobody sees, nobody knows, or a God known?

The Impersonal God is a living God, a Principle.
The difference between Personal and Impersonal God
is this: the Personal God is only a man, whereas the
Impersonal is angel, man, animal, and yet something
more, which we cannot see, because impersonality
includes all personalities, is the sum total of everything
in the universe, and infinitely more besides. "As the
one fire coming into the world manifests itself in so
many forms, and yet is infinitely more besides"—even
so is the Impersonal.

We want to worship a living God. I have not seen
anything but God all my life, nor have you. To see
this chair you must first see God and then the chair,
in and through Him. He is everywhere, as the "I am."
The moment you feel "I am," you are conscious of
Existence. Where shall we find God if we cannot see
Him in our own hearts and in every living being?
"Thou art the man, Thou art the woman, Thou art
the girl, and Thou art the boy; Thou art the old man
tottering with a stick, Thou art the young man walking in the pride of his strength; Thou art all that ex-

ists"—a wonderful, living God who is the only fact in the universe.

This seems to many to be a terrible contradiction of the traditional God, who lives behind a veil somewhere and whom nobody ever sees. The priests only give us an assurance that if we follow them, listen to their admonitions, and walk in the way they mark out for us, then, when we die, they will give us a passport to enable us to see the face of God! What are all these ideas of heaven but simply inventions of this nonsensical priestcraft?

Of course, the idea of the Impersonal is very destructive: it takes away all trade from the priests, churches, and temples. In India there is a famine now, but there are temples in each one of which there are jewels worth a king's ransom. If the priests taught this idea of the Impersonal to the people, their occupation would be gone. Yet we have to teach it unselfishly, without priestcraft. You are God and so am I. Who obeys whom? Who worships whom? You are the highest temple of God; I would rather worship you than any temple, image, or Bible. Why are some people's thoughts so full of contradictions? They say that they are hard-headed practical men. Very good. But what is more practical than worshipping you? I see you, feel you, and I know you are God. The Mohammedan says there is no God but Allah. Vedānta says there is nothing that is not God. It may frighten many of you, but you will understand it by degrees. The living God is within you, and yet you are building churches and temples and believing all sorts of imaginary nonsense. The only God to

worship is the human soul in the human body. Of
course, all animals are temples too, but man is the
highest, the greatest of all temples. If I cannot
worship in that, no other temple will be of any
advantage. The moment I have realized God sitting
in the temple of every human body, the moment
I stand in reverence before every human being and
see God in him, that moment I am free from
bondage, everything that binds vanishes, and I am
free.

This is the most practical of all worship; it has
nothing to do with theorizing and speculation. Yet it
frightens many. They say it is not right. They go on
theorizing about old ideas told them by their grandfathers, that a God somewhere in heaven had told
someone that he was God. Since that time we have
had only theories. This is practicality according to
them—and our ideas are impractical! No doubt,
Vedānta says, each one must have his own path;
but the path is not the goal. The worship of a God
in heaven and all these things are not bad; but they
are only steps towards the Truth, and not the Truth
itself. They are good and beautiful, and some wonderful ideas are there, but Vedānta says at every point:
"My friend, Him whom you are worshipping as
unknown—I worship Him as you. He whom you
are worshipping as unknown and are seeking throughout the universe has been with you all the time. You
are living through Him and He is the eternal Witness
of the universe." He whom all the Vedas worship,
nay more, He who is always present in the eternal
"I"—He existing, the whole universe exists. He is the

light and life of the universe. If this "I" were not in you, you would not see the sun; everything would be a mass of darkness. He shining, you see the world.

One objection is generally raised, and it is this: that this may lead to a tremendous amount of difficulty. Every one of us will think, "I am God, and whatever I do or think must be good; for God can do no evil." In the first place, even taking this danger of misinterpretation for granted, can it be proved that on the other side the same danger does not exist? Men have been worshipping a God in heaven separate from them and of whom they are much afraid. They have been born shaking with fear, and all their life they will go on shaking. Has the world been made much better by this? Those who have understood and worshipped a Personal God, and those who have understood and worshipped an Impersonal God—which of these have been the great workers of the world? On which side have been the gigantic workers, gigantic moral powers? Certainly on the side of the Impersonal. How can you expect morality to be developed through fear? It can never be. "When one sees another, when one hears another, that is māyā. When one does not see another, when one does not hear another, when everything has become Ātman, who sees whom, who perceives whom?" It is all He and all I at the same time. The soul has become pure. Then and then alone do we understand what love is. Love cannot come through fear. Its basis is freedom. When we really begin to love the world, then we understand what is meant by the brotherhood of mankind, and not before.

So it is not right to say that the idea of the Impersonal will lead to a tremendous amount of evil in the world, as if the other doctrine never lent itself to works of evil; as if it did not lead to sectarianism, deluging the world with blood and causing men to tear each other to pieces. "My God is the greatest God; if anyone disagrees, let us decide it by a free fight"—that is the outcome of dualism all over the world. Come out into the broad, open light of day; come out from the little narrow paths. For how can the infinite Soul rest content to live and die in small ruts? Come out into the universe of light. Everything in the universe is yours. Stretch out your arms and embrace it with love. If you ever felt you wanted to do that, you have felt God.

You remember that passage in the sermon of Buddha: how he sent a thought of love towards the south, the north, the east, and the west, above and below, until the whole universe was filled with this love, so grand, great, and infinite. When you have that feeling you have true personality; for the whole universe is one Person. Let little things go. Give up the small for the Infinite; give up small enjoyments for Infinite Bliss. It is all yours, for the Impersonal includes the personal. So God is personal and impersonal at the same time. And Man—the infinite Impersonal Man—is manifesting Himself as a person. We, the Infinite, have limited ourselves, as it were, into small parts.

Vedānta says that infinity is our true nature; it will never vanish; it will abide for ever. But we limit ourselves by our karma, which like a chain round our necks has dragged us into this limitation. Break that chain and be free. Trample law under your feet. No law can bind man's true nature—no destiny, no fate. How can there be law in infinity? Freedom is its watchword. Freedom is its nature, its birthright. Be free and then have any number of personalities you like. Then we shall play like the actor who comes upon the stage and plays the part of a beggar. Contrast him with the actual beggar walking in the streets. The scene is perhaps the same in both cases; the words are perhaps the same; but yet what a difference! The one enjoys his beggary, while the other is suffering misery from it. And what makes this difference? The one is free and the other is bound. The actor knows that his beggary is not true, but that he has assumed it for the play, while the real beggar thinks that it is his own natural state and he has to bear it whether he will or not; for this is the law.

So long as we have no knowledge of our real nature, we are beggars, jostled about by every force in nature and made slaves of by everything in nature. We cry all over the world for help, but help never comes to us. We cry to imaginary beings and yet it never comes. But still we hope help will come; and thus in weeping, wailing, and hoping, this life is passed and the same play goes on and on.

Be free. Hope for nothing from anyone. I am sure if you look back upon your lives you will find that you were always vainly trying to get help from others which never came. All the help that ever came was from within yourselves. You had the fruits only of what you yourselves worked for, and yet you were strangely hoping all the time for help from others.

A rich man's parlour is always full; but, if you notice, you do not find the same people there. The visitors are always hoping that they will get something from the wealthy man; but they never do. So are our lives spent in hoping, hoping, hoping, to which there is no end. Give up hope, says Vedānta. Why should you hope? You *have* everything, nay, you *are* everything. What are you hoping for? If a king goes mad and runs about trying to find the king of his country, he will never find him, because he is the king himself. He may go through every village and city in his own country, seeking in every house, weeping and wailing, but he will never find him, because he is the king himself. It is better that we know we are God and give up this fool's search after Him. Knowing we are God, we become happy and contented.

Give up all these mad pursuits and then play your part in the universe as an actor on the stage. The whole scene will change, and instead of an eternal prison this world will appear a playground; instead of a land of competition it will be a land of bliss, where perpetual spring exists, flowers bloom, and butterflies flit about. This very world, which formerly was a hell, will be a heaven. To the eyes of the bound it is a tremendous place of torment, but to the eyes of the free it is quite otherwise. This very life is the Universal Life. Heavens and all those places are here; all the gods are here, the so-called prototypes of man. The gods did not create man after their image, but man created the gods. And here are the prototypes; here is Indra, here is Varuna, and all the gods of the universe. We have been projecting our little doubles, and we are the originals of these gods; we are the real, the only gods to be worshipped.

This is the view of Vedānta, and this is its practicality. When we have become free, we need not go crazy and give up society and rush off to die in the forest or in a cave. We shall remain where we are, only we shall understand the whole thing. The same phenomena will remain, but with a new meaning.

We do not know the world yet; it is only through freedom that we shall see what it is and understand its nature. We shall see then that this so-called law, or fate, or destiny, touched only a small fraction of our nature. It was only one side, but on the other side there was freedom all the time. We did not know this, and that is why we tried to save ourselves from evil by hiding our faces in the ground, like hunted hares. Through delusion we tried to forget our nature, and yet we could not; it was always calling to us, and all our search after God or the gods or external freedom was a search after our real nature. We mistook the voice. We thought it came from the fire or from a god, or from the sun or moon or stars. But at last we have found that it is from within ourselves. Within ourselves is this eternal voice speaking of eternal freedom; its music is eternally going on. Part of this music of the Soul has become the earth, the law, this universe; but it was always ours and always will be.

In one word, the ideal of Vedānta is to know man as he really is; and this is its message: If you cannot worship your brother man, the manifested God, how can you worship a God who is unmanifested? Do you not remember what the Bible says: "If you cannot love

your brother whom you have seen, how can you love
God whom you have not seen?" If you cannot see
God in the human face, how can you see Him in the
clouds or in images made of dull, dead matter, or in
the mere fictions of your brain? I shall call you
religious from the day you begin to see God in men
and women. Then you will understand what is meant
by turning the left cheek to the man who strikes you
on the right. When you see man as God, everything,
even the tiger, will be welcome. Whatever comes to
us is but the Lord, the Eternal, the Blessed One,
appearing to us in various forms—as our father and
mother and friend and child. They are our own Soul
playing with us.

As our human relationships can thus be made
divine, so our relationship with God may take any
of these forms, and we can look upon Him as our
Father or Mother or Friend or Beloved. Calling God
Mother is a higher ideal than calling God Father, and
to call Him Friend is still higher; but the highest is
to regard Him as the Beloved. The culmination of all
is to see no difference between lover and beloved.
You may remember, perhaps, the old Persian story of
how a lover came and knocked at the door of his
beloved and was asked, "Who are you?" He answered,
"It is I," and there was no response. A second time he
came and exclaimed, "I am here," but the door was
not opened. A third time he came, and the voice asked
from inside, "Who is there?" He replied, "I am thyself,
my beloved," and the door opened. So is the relation
between God and ourselves. He is in everything; He
is everything. Every man and woman is the palpable,

blissful, living God. Who says God is unknown? Who says He is to be searched after? We have known God eternally. We have been living in Him eternally. Everywhere He is eternally known, eternally worshipped.

Then comes another idea: that other forms of worship are not errors. This is one of the great points to be remembered: that those who worship God through ceremonials and forms, however crude we may think them, are not in error. It is the journey from truth to truth, from lower truth to higher truth. Darkness means less light; evil means less good; impurity means less purity. It must always be borne in mind that we should see others with eyes of love, with sympathy, knowing that they are going along the same path that we have trodden. If you are free, you must know that all will be so sooner or later; if you are free, how can you see anyone in bondage? If you are really pure, how do you see the impure? For what is within is without. We cannot see impurity without having it inside ourselves.

This is one of the practical sides of Vedānta, and I hope that we shall all try to carry it into our lives. Our whole life here is an opportunity to carry this into practice. But our greatest gain is that we shall work with satisfaction and contentment instead of with discontent and dissatisfaction; for we know that Truth is within us, we have It as our birthright, and we have only to manifest It and make It tangible.

PRACTICAL VEDĀNTA

PART III

(Delivered in London, November 17, 1896)

IN THE *Chhāndogya Upanishad* we read that a sage named Nārada comes to another named Sanatkumāra and asks him various questions, one of which is concerning the cause of things as they are. And Sanatkumāra leads him, as it were, step by step, telling him that there is something higher than this earth and something higher than that, and so on, till he comes to ākāśa. Ākāśa is higher than light, because in ākāśa exist the sun and the moon, lightning, and the stars; in ākāśa we live and in ākāśa we die. Then the question arises whether there is anything higher than that, and Sanatkumāra tells him of prāna. This prāna, according to Vedānta, is the principle of life. It is, like ākāśa, an omnipresent principle; and all motion, either in the body or anywhere else, is the work of prāna. It is higher than ākāśa, and through it everything lives. Prāna is in the mother, in the father, in the sister, in the teacher; prāna is the knower.

I will read another passage, where Śvetaketu asks his father about Truth. The father teaches him different things and concludes by saying: "That which is the subtle cause of all these things—of It are all these things made. That is the All; That is Truth. Thou art That, O Śvetaketu." And then he gives various

252

examples: "As a bee, O Śvetaketu, gathers honey from different flowers, and as the different honeys do not know that they come from various trees and from various flowers, so all of us, having come from that Existence, know not that we have done so. Now, That which is that subtle essence—in It all that exists has its Self. It is the True; It is the Self. And thou, O Śvetaketu, art That." He gives another example, of the rivers running down to the ocean: "As rivers coming from various sources ultimately flow into the ocean but do not know where they have come from, even so, though we have come out of that Existence, we do not know that we are That. O Śvetaketu, thou art That." So he goes on with his teachings.

Now, there are two principles of knowledge. The one principle is that we can know only by referring the particular to the general, and the general to the universal; and the second is that anything of which the explanation is sought, is to be explained as far as possible from its own nature. Taking up the first principle, we see that all our knowledge really consists of classifications, going higher and higher. When something happens once, we are, as it were, dissatisfied. When it can be shown that the same thing happens again and again, we are satisfied and call it law. When we find that one apple falls, we are dissatisfied; but when we find that all apples fall, we call it the law of gravitation and are satisfied. The fact is that from the particular we deduce the general.

When we want to study religion, we should apply this scientific process. The same principle also holds good here; and as a matter of fact we find that that has been the method throughout. In reading these books from which I have been translating to you, the earliest idea that I can trace is this principle of going from the particular to the general. We see how the gods, the "bright ones," become merged into a principle; and likewise, in their ideas of the cosmos, we find the ancient thinkers going higher and higher—from the fine elements they go to finer and more embracing elements, and from these particulars they come to one omnipresent ākāśa, and even from that they go to an all-embracing force, or prāna. And through all this runs the principle that one is not separate from the others. It is the very ākāśa that exists in the higher form of prāna; or the higher form of prāna is con-cretized, so to say, and becomes ākāśa, and that ākāśa becomes still grosser, and so on.

The generalization of the Personal God is another case in point. We have seen how this generalization was reached, and how the Personal God was called the sum total of all consciousness. But a difficulty arises: it is an incomplete generalization. We take up only one side of the facts of nature, the fact of consciousness, and upon that we generalize; but the other side, namely, inert nature, is left out. So in the first place it is a defective generalization.

There is another insufficiency about the Personal God, and it relates to the second principle, namely, that everything should be explained from its own nature. There may have been people who ascribed the falling of apples to ghosts; but the scientific explanation is the law of gravitation. And although we know it is not a perfect explanation, yet it is much better than the other, because it is derived from the nature of the thing itself, while the other posits an extraneous cause. So throughout the whole range of our knowledge: the explanation which is based upon the nature of the thing itself is a scientific explanation, and the explanation which brings in an outside agent is unscientific.

So the explanation of a Personal God as the Creator of the universe has to stand that test. If that God is said to be outside nature, having nothing to do with nature, and if nature is said to be the outcome of the command of that God and to have been produced from nothing, then it is a very unscientific theory. This has been the weak point of every theistic religion throughout the ages. These two defects we find in what is generally called the theory of monotheism, the theory of a Personal God, endowed with all the qualities of a human being multiplied very much, who by His will created this universe out of nothing and yet is separate from it.

This, as we have seen, leads us into two difficulties: It is not a sufficient generalization, and secondly, it is not an explanation of nature from within itself. It holds that the effect is not the cause, that the cause is entirely separate from the effect. Yet all human knowledge shows that the effect is but the cause in another form. To this idea the discoveries of modern science are tending every day, and the latest theory, which has been accepted on all sides, is the theory of evolution, the principle of which is that the effect is but the cause in another form, a readjustment of the cause, and that the cause takes the form of the effect. The theory of creation out of nothing would be laughed at by modern scientists.

Now, can religion stand these tests? If there be any religious theories which can stand these two tests, they will be acceptable to the modern mind, to the thinking mind. Any other theory which we ask the modern man to believe—on the authority of priests or churches or books—he is unable to accept, and the result is a hideous mass of unbelief. Even those in whom there is an external display of belief have in their hearts a tremendous amount of unbelief. The rest of the people shrink away from religion; they give it up, regarding it as priestcraft only.

Religion in modern times has been reduced to a sort of national affair: It is one of our very best social remnants; so let it remain. But the real need which our grandfathers felt for it is gone; we no longer find it satisfactory to our reason. The idea of such a Personal God and such a creation, the idea generally known as monotheism in every religion, cannot hold its own any longer. In India it could not hold its own because of the Buddhists; and that was the very point where they gained their victory in ancient times. They showed that if we admit that nature is possessed of infinite power, and that nature can work out all its wants, it is simply unnecessary to insist that there is something besides nature. Even the soul is unnecessary.

The discussion about substance and qualities is very old, and you will sometimes find that the old superstition lives even at the present day. Most of you have read how, during the middle ages, and, I am sorry to say, even much later, this was one of the subjects of discussion: whether qualities inhere in substance, whether length, breadth, and thickness inhere in the substance which we call dead matter, or whether the substance can exist whether the qualities are there or not. To this our Buddhist says: "You have no ground for maintaining the existence of such a substance. The qualities are all that exist. You do not see beyond them." This is just the position of most of our modern agnostics. For it is this fight about substance and qualities that, on a higher plane, takes the form of the fight about noumenon and phenomenon. There is the phenomenal world, the universe of continuous change, and there is something behind which does not change; and this duality of existence— noumenon and phenomenon—some hold to be real, while others, with better reason, claim that you have no right to admit the two, for what we see, feel, and think of is only the phenomenon. You have no right, they say, to assert that there is anything beyond the phenomenon; and apparently there has been no answer to this.

But the monistic school of Vedānta has given the answer. According to it, one thing alone exists, and that one thing is either phenomenon or noumenon. It is not true that there are two: something changing, and, in and through that, something which does not change; but it is one and the same thing which appears as changing and is in reality unchangeable. We have come to think of the body and mind and soul as separate, but really there is only one; and that one appears through these various forms. Take the well-known illustration of the monists: the rope appearing as the snake. Some people, in the dark or for some other reason, mistake a rope for a snake; but when knowledge comes, the snake vanishes and it is found to be a rope. By this illustration we see that when the snake exists in the mind, the rope has vanished, and when the rope exists, the snake has gone. When we see the phenomenon, and the phenomenon only, around us, the noumenon has vanished; but when we see the noumenon, the unchangeable, it naturally follows that the phenomenon has vanished.

Now we understand better the position of both the realist and the idealist. The realist sees the phenomenon only, and the idealist looks at the noumenon. For the idealist, the really genuine idealist, who has truly acquired that power of perception whereby he can get away from all ideas of change—for him the changeful universe has vanished, and he has the right to say that it is all delusion and there is no change. The realist, at the same time, looks at the changeful phenomenon. For him the unchangeable has vanished, and he has the right to say that the phenomenon alone is real.

What is the outcome of this discussion? It is that the idea of a Personal God is not sufficient. We have to get to something higher, to the idea of the Impersonal. It is the only logical step that we can take. Not that the idea of the Personal God will be destroyed by that, not that we have proved that the Personal God does not exist; but we must go to the Impersonal for the explanation of the Personal God, for the Impersonal is a much higher generalization. Only the Impersonal can be infinite; the Personal is limited. Thus we preserve the Personal God and do not destroy Him. Often the doubt comes to us that if we hold to the idea of the Impersonal God, the Personal God may be destroyed; if we hold to the idea of the Impersonal Man, the personal man may be lost. But the Vedāntic idea is not the destruction of the individual, but its real vindication. We cannot prove the existence of the individual except by referring to the universal, by proving that the individual is really the universal. If we think of the individual as separate from everything else in the universe, it cannot stand a minute. Such a thing never existed.

Secondly, by the application of the other principle, that the explanation of everything must come out of the nature of the thing, we are led to a still bolder idea and one more difficult to understand. It is nothing less than this: The Impersonal Being, our highest generalization, is in ourselves and we are That. "O Śvetaketu, thou art That." You are that Impersonal Being; that God for whom you searched all over the universe has been all the time you yourself—yourself not in the personal sense but in the impersonal. The man we know now, the manifested, is personalized, but the reality in him is the Impersonal. To understand the personal we have to refer it to the Impersonal; the particular must be referred to the general. And that Impersonal is the true Self of man.

There will be various questions in connexion with this, and I shall try to answer them as we go on. Many difficulties will arise. But first let us clearly understand the position of monism. As manifested beings we appear to be separate, but our reality is One, and the less we think of ourselves as separate from that One, the better for us. The more we think of ourselves as separate from the whole, the more miserable we become.

From this monistic principle we get at the basis of ethics, and I venture to say that we cannot get any ethics from anywhere else. We know that the oldest idea of ethics was that it was based on the will of some particular being or beings; but few are ready to accept that now, because it would be only a partial generalization. The Hindus say we must not do this and must do that because the Vedas say so; but the Christian is not going to obey the authority of the Vedas. The Christian says you must do this and not do that because the Bible says so. That will not be binding on those who do not believe in the Bible. But we must have a theory which is large enough to take in all these various viewpoints. Just as there are millions of people who are ready to believe in a Personal Creator, there have also been thousands of the brightest minds in this world who have felt that such ideas were not sufficient for them and wanted something higher; and wherever religion was not broad enough to include all these minds, the result was that the brightest minds in society remained outside religion. Never was this so marked as at the present time, especially in Europe.

Therefore religion must become broad enough to include these minds. Everything it claims must be judged from the standpoint of reason. Why religions should claim that they are not bound to abide by reason no one knows. If one does not take the standard of reason there cannot be any true judgement, even in religion. One religion may ordain something very hideous. For instance, the Mohammedan religion allows Mohammedans to kill all who are not of their religion. It is clearly stated in the Koran: "Kill the infidels if they do not become Mohammedans." They must be put to fire and sword. Now, if we tell a Mohammedan that this is wrong, he will naturally ask: "How do you know that? How do you know it is not good? My book says it is." If you point out that your book is older, the Buddhist will come and say, "My book is much older still." Then will come the Hindu and say, "My books are the oldest of all." Therefore referring to books will not do. Where is the standard by which you can compare? You will say, "Look at the Sermon on the Mount," and the Mohammedan will reply, "Look at the ethics of the Koran." The Mohammedan will say, "Who is the arbiter as to which is the better of the two?" Neither the New Testament nor the Koran can be the arbiter in a quarrel between them. There must be some independent authority, and that cannot be any book, but something that is universal. And what is more universal than reason?

It has been said that reason is not always strong enough to help us to get at the truth; many times it makes mistakes; and therefore the conclusion is that we must believe in the authority of a church! That was said to me by a Roman Catholic, but I could not see the logic of it. On the other hand, I should say, if reason is so weak, a body of priests would be weaker, and I am not going to accept their verdict, but I will abide by my reason, because with all its weakness there is some chance of my getting at the truth through it, while by the other means there is no such hope at all.

We should therefore follow reason, and also we should sympathize with those who, following reason, do not come to any sort of belief. For it is better that mankind should become atheists by following reason than blindly believe in two hundred millions of gods on the authority of somebody. What we want is progress, development, realization. No theories ever made men higher. No amount of books can help us to become purer. The only power is in realization, and that lies in ourselves and comes from thinking. Let men think. A clod of earth never thinks; but it remains only a clod of earth. The glory of man is that he is a thinking being. It is the nature of man to think, and therein he differs from animals. I believe in reason and follow reason, having seen enough of the evils of authority; for I was born in a country where people have gone to the extreme in authority.

The Hindus believe that creation has come out of the Vedas. How do you know there is a cow? Because the word cow is in the Vedas. How do you know there is a man? Because the word man is there. If it had not been, there would have been no man in the world. That is what they say. Authority with a vengeance! Some of the most powerful minds have taken this idea up and spun out wonderful logical theories round it. They have reasoned it out, and there it stands, a whole system of philosophy; and thousands of the brightest intellects have been dedicated through hundreds of years to the working out of this idea. Such has been the power of authority, and great are the dangers thereof. It stunts the growth of humanity, and we must not forget that we want growth. In all our attempts to find out relative truth, what we want, even more than the truth itself, is the exercise of the mind. That exercise is, indeed, our life.

The monistic theory has this merit: It is the most rational of all the religious theories that we can conceive of. Every other theory, every conception of God which is partial and petty and personal, is not rational. And yet monism is so grand that it embraces all these partial conceptions of God as being necessary for many. Some people say that though this personal explanation is irrational, it is consoling. They want a consoling religion, and we understand that it is necessary for them. The clear light of truth very few in this life can bear, much less live up to. It is necessary, therefore, that this comfortable religion should exist; it helps many souls to find a better one. Small minds, whose circumference is very limited and who require little things to build them up, never venture to soar high in thought. Their conceptions, even if only of little gods and symbols, are very good and helpful to them.

But you have to understand the Impersonal, for it is in and through That alone that these others can be explained. Take, for instance, the idea of the Personal God. A man who understands and believes in the Impersonal—John Stuart Mill, for example—may say that a Personal God is impossible and cannot be proved. I agree with him that a Personal God cannot

be demonstrated. But He is the highest reading of the
Impersonal that can be reached by the human intellect;
and what else is the universe but various readings of
the Absolute? It is like a book before us, and each
one has brought his intellect to read It, and each one
has to read It for himself. There is something which
is common to the intellects of all men; therefore certain
things appear to be the same to all. That you and I
see a chair proves there is something common to both
our minds. If a being comes with another sense, he
will not see the chair at all. But all beings similarly
constituted will see the same things. Thus this universe
itself is the Absolute, the Unchangeable, the noumenon; and the reading thereof constitutes the phenomenon. For you will find that all phenomena are
finite; every phenomenon that we can see, feel, or
think of is finite, limited by our knowledge. And the
Personal God, as we conceive of Him, is in fact a
phenomenon. The very idea of causation exists only
in the phenomenal world, and God as the cause of this
universe must naturally be thought of as limited; and
yet He is the same Impersonal God. This phenomenal
universe, as we have seen, is the same Impersonal
Being read by our intellect. Whatever is real in the
universe is that Impersonal Being, and the forms and
names are given by our intellects. Whatever is real
in this table is that Being, and the table form and all
else are given by our intellects.

Now, motion, for instance, which is a necessary
adjunct of the phenomenal, cannot be predicated of the
universal. Every particle, every atom in the universe,
is in a constant state of change and motion, but the

universe as a whole is unchangeable, because motion
or change is a relative thing; we can think of something
in motion only in comparison with something which
is not moving. There must be two things in order to
understand motion. The whole mass of the universe,
taken as a unit, cannot move. In regard to what will it
move? It cannot be said to change. In regard to what
will it change? So the whole is the Absolute; but
within It every particle is in a constant state of flux
and change. It is unchangeable and changeable at the
same time, impersonal and personal in one. This is
our conception of the universe, of motion, and of God.

Thus we see that the Impersonal, instead of doing
away with the Personal—the Absolute, instead of
pulling down the relative—only explains it to the full
satisfaction of our reason and heart. The Personal God
and all that exists in the universe are the same Impersonal Being seen through our minds. When we shall
be rid of our minds, our little personalities, we shall
become one with It. This is what is meant by "Thou
art That." We must know our true nature, the
Absolute.

The finite, manifested man forgets his source and
thinks himself to be an entirely separate entity. We,
as personalized, differentiated beings, forget our reality,
and the teaching of monism is not that we must give
up these differentiations, but that we must learn to
understand what they are. We are in reality that
Infinite Being, and our personalities represent so many
channels through which this Infinite Reality is manifesting Itself; and the whole mass of changes which
we call evolution is brought about by the soul's trying

to manifest more and more of its infinite energy. We cannot stop anywhere on this side of the Infinite; our power and blessedness and wisdom cannot but grow into the Infinite. Infinite power and existence and blessedness are ours, and we do not have to acquire them; they are our own and we have only to manifest them.

This is the central idea of monism, and one that is very hard to understand. From my childhood everyone around me taught me weakness; I have been told ever since I was born that I was a weak thing. It is very difficult for me now to realize my own strength; but by analysis and reasoning I gain knowledge of my own strength, I realize it. All the knowledge that we have in this world—where does it come from? It is within us. What knowledge is outside? None. Knowledge is not in matter; it is in man all the time. Nobody ever creates knowledge; man brings it from within. It is lying there. The whole of the big banyan tree which covers acres of ground is in a little seed which is perhaps no bigger than one-eighth of a mustard seed; all that mass of energy is confined there. The gigantic intellect, we know, lies coiled up in the protoplasmic cell; and why should not infinite energy? We know that it is so. It may seem like a paradox, but it is true. Each one of us comes out of a protoplasmic cell, and all the powers we possess are coiled up there. You cannot say they come from food; for if you heap up food mountain high, what power comes out of it? The energy is in the cell, potentially no doubt, but still there.

So infinite power is in the soul of man, whether he

knows it or not. Its manifestation is only a question of being conscious of it. Slowly this infinite giant is, as it were, waking up, becoming conscious of his power, and arousing himself; and with his growing consciousness, more and more of his bonds are breaking, his chains are bursting asunder, and the day is sure to come when, with the full consciousness of his infinite power and wisdom, the giant will rise to his feet and stand erect. Let us all help to hasten that glorious consummation.

PRACTICAL VEDĀNTA

PART IV

(Delivered in London, November 18, 1896)

SO FAR WE HAVE BEEN DEALING mostly with the universal. This morning I shall try to place before you the Vedāntic ideas of the relation of the particular to the universal. As we have seen, in the earlier, dualistic form of the Vedic doctrines, there was a clearly defined particular and limited soul for every being. There have been a great many theories about this particular soul in each individual, but the main discussion was between the ancient Vedāntists and the ancient Buddhists, the former believing in the individual soul as complete in itself, the latter denying *in toto* the existence of such an individual soul. As I told you the other day, it is pretty much the same discussion you have in Europe as to substance and qualities, one party holding that behind the qualities there is something known as substance, in which the qualities inhere, and the other denying the existence of such a substance, as being unnecessary, for the qualities may exist by themselves.

The most ancient theory of the soul, of course, is based upon the argument of self-identity—"I am I": that the "I" of yesterday is the "I" of today, and the "I" of today will be the "I" of tomorrow; that in spite of all the changes that are happening to the body,

I yet believe that I am the same "I." This seems to have been the central argument with those who believed in a limited, and yet perfectly complete, individual soul.

On the other hand, the ancient Buddhists denied the necessity of such an assumption. They brought forward the argument that all that we know and all that we possibly can know are simply these changes. The positing of an unchangeable and unchanging substance is simply superfluous, and even if there were any such unchangeable thing, we could never understand it, nor should we ever be able to cognize it in any sense of the word.

The same discussion you will find going on at the present time in Europe between the religionists and the idealists on the one side, and the modern positivists and agnostics on the other—one set believing that there is something which does not change (of whom the latest representative is your Herbert Spencer), and that we catch a glimpse of something which is unchangeable; and the other being represented by the modern Comtists and modern agnostics. Those of you who were interested a few years ago in the discussions between Herbert Spencer and Frederick Harrison might have noticed that it was the same old difficulty, the one party standing for a substance behind the changeful, and the other party denying the necessity for such an assumption. One party says we cannot conceive of changes without conceiving of something which does not change. The other party brings out the argument that this is superfluous; we can only conceive of something which changes, and as to the unchanging, we can neither know, feel, nor sense it.

In India this great question did not find its solution in very ancient times, because, as we have seen, the assumption of a substance behind the qualities which is not the qualities can never be substantiated. Nay, even the argument from self-identity, from memory— that I am the "I" of yesterday because I remember it, and therefore I have been a continuous something— cannot be substantiated. The other quibble that is generally put forward is a mere delusion of words. For instance, a man may take a long series of such sentences as "I do," "I go," "I dream," "I sleep," "I move," and here you will find it claimed that the doing, going, dreaming, and so forth, have been changing, but what remained constant was that "I." Therefore they conclude that the "I" is something constant, and an individual in itself, but all these changes belong to the body. This, though apparently very convincing and clear, is based upon mere play on words. The "I" and the doing, going, and dreaming may be separate in black and white, but no one can separate them in his mind. When I eat, I think of myself as eating—I am identified with eating. When I run, I and the running are not two separate things. Thus the argument from personal identity does not seem to be very strong.

The other argument, the argument from memory, is also weak. If the identity of my being is represented by my memory, then it will have to be admitted that I did not exist at those times which I have forgotten. And we know that people under certain conditions forget their whole past. In many cases of lunacy a man thinks of himself as made of glass or as being an animal. If the existence of that man depended on his memory, then he should have been made of glass—which not being so, we cannot make the identity of the self depend on such a flimsy thing as memory. Thus we see that the soul as a limited, yet complete and continuing identity cannot be established as separate from qualities. We cannot establish a narrowed-down, limited existence to which is attached a bundle of qualities.

On the other hand, the argument of the ancient Buddhists seems to be stronger—that we do not know, and cannot know, anything that is beyond this bundle of qualities. According to them the soul consists of certain qualities called sensations and feelings. An aggregate of these is what is called the soul, and this aggregate is continually changing.

The Advaitist theory of the soul reconciles both these positions. The position of the Advaitist is that it is true that we cannot think of the substance as separate from the qualities; we cannot think of change and not-change at the same time. It would be impossible. But the very thing which is called the substance is also the qualities; substance and qualities are not two things. It is the unchangeable that is appearing as the changeable. The unchangeable substance of the universe is not something separate from it. The noumenon is not something different from the phenomenon, but it is the very noumenon which has become the phenomenon. There is a Soul, which is unchanging, and what we call feelings and perceptions, nay, even the body, are that very Soul seen from another point of view. We have got into the habit of thinking that we have bodies and souls, and so forth, but properly speaking, there is only one. When I think of myself as the body, I am only a body; it is meaningless to say I am something else. And when I think of myself as the Soul, the body vanishes; the perception of the body does not remain. None can have the perception of the Soul unless his perception of the body has vanished; none can have the perception of the substance unless his perception of the qualities has vanished.

The ancient illustration of Advaita, of a rope being taken for a snake, may elucidate the point a little more. When a man mistakes the rope for a snake, the rope has vanished, and when he takes it for a rope, the snake has vanished and only the rope remains. The ideas of dual or treble existence come from reasoning on insufficient data, and we read of them in books or hear about them until we come under the delusion that we really have a dual perception of the Soul and the body; but such a perception never really exists. The perception is either of the body or of the Soul. It requires no arguments to prove it; you can verify it in your own minds.

Try to think of yourself as the Soul, as something disembodied. You will find it to be almost impossible, and those few who are able to do so will find that at the time when they realize themselves as the Soul they have no idea of the body. You have heard of, or perhaps have seen, persons who on particular occasions have been in peculiar states of mind brought about by deep meditation, self-hypnotism, hysteria, or drugs. From their experience you may gather that when they were perceiving something internally, the external had vanished for them. This shows that whatever exists is one. That unity is appearing in these various forms, and all these various forms give rise to the relation of cause and effect. The relation of cause and effect is one of evolution—the one becomes the other, and so on. Sometimes the cause vanishes, as it were, and in its place leaves the effect. If the Soul is the cause of the body, the Soul, as it were, vanishes for the time being and the body remains, and when the body vanishes, the Soul remains. This theory meets the arguments of the Buddhists that were levelled against the assumption of the dualism of body and Soul, by denying the duality and showing that the substance and the qualities are one and the same thing appearing in various forms.

We have also seen that this idea of the unchangeable can be established only as regards the whole, but never as regards the part. The very idea of parts comes from the idea of change or motion. Everything that is limited we can understand and know, because it is changeable; and the whole must be unchangeable, because there is no other thing besides it in relation to which change would be possible. Change is always in regard to something which does not change, or which changes relatively less. According to Advaita, therefore, the idea of the Soul as universal, unchangeable, and immortal can be demonstrated. The difficulty would be as regards the particular. What shall we do with the old dualistic theories, which have such a hold upon us and which we all have to pass through—these beliefs in limited, little, individual souls?

We have seen that we are immortal as the whole; but the difficulty is that we desire so much to be immortal as *parts* of the whole. We have seen that we are the Infinite, and that That is our real individuality; but we want so much to make these little souls individual. What becomes of them when we find in our everyday experience that these little souls are individuals with only the reservation that they are continuously growing individuals? They are the same, yet not the same. The "I" of yesterday is the "I" of today, and yet not so; it is changed somewhat.

Now, by getting rid of the dualistic conception that in the midst of all these changes there is something that does not change, and taking the most modern of conceptions, that of evolution, we find that the "I" is a continuously changing, expanding entity. If it be true that man is the evolution of a mollusc, the mollusc individual is the same as the man, only it has become expanded a great deal. From mollusc to man it has been a continuous expansion towards infinity. Therefore the limited soul can be styled an individual who is continuously expanding towards the Infinite Individual. Perfect individuality will be reached only when it has reached the Infinite, but on this side of the Infinite it is a continuously changing, growing personality.

One of the remarkable features of the Advaita system of Vedānta is that it harmonized the preceding systems. Our ancient philosophers knew what you call the theory of evolution—that growth is gradual, step by step; and the recognition of this led them to harmonize all the preceding systems. Thus not one of these preceding steps was rejected. The fault of the Buddhist faith was that it had neither the faculty nor the perception of this continual, expansive growth, and for this reason it never even made an attempt to harmonize itself with the pre-existing steps towards the ideal. They were rejected as useless and harmful.

This tendency in religion is itself most harmful. A man gets a new and better idea and then he looks back on those he has given up, and forthwith decides that they were mischievous and unnecessary. He never thinks that, however crude they may appear from his present point of view, they were very useful to him, that they were necessary if he was to reach his present state, and that every one of us has to grow in a similar fashion, living first on crude ideas, deriving benefit from them, and then arriving at a higher standard. With the oldest theories, therefore, Advaita is friendly. Dualism and all the systems that preceded it are accepted by Advaita, not in a patronizing way, but with the conviction that they are true, being manifestations of the same Truth, and that they all lead to the same conclusion that Advaita has reached.

With blessings, and not with curses, should be preserved all these various steps through which humanity had to pass. Therefore all these dualistic systems have never been rejected or thrown out, but have been kept intact in Vedānta, and the dualistic conception of an individual soul, limited, yet complete in itself, finds its place in Vedānta. According to dualism man dies and goes to other worlds, and so forth, and

these ideas are kept in Vedānta in their entirety. For
with the recognition of growth, in the Advaita system,
these theories are given their proper place by admitting
that they represent only a partial view of Truth.

From the dualistic standpoint this universe can only
be looked upon as a creation of matter or force, can
only be looked upon as the play of a certain will; and
that will, again, can only be looked upon as separate
from the universe. Thus, from such a standpoint, a
man has to see himself as composed of a dual nature
—body and soul; and this soul, though limited, is
individually complete in itself. Such a man's ideas of
immortality and of the future life will necessarily
accord with his idea of the soul. These phases have
been kept in Vedānta, and it is therefore necessary for
me to present to you a few of the popular ideas of
dualism.

According to this theory we have a body, of course,
and behind the body there is what is called a fine body.
This fine body is also made of matter, only very fine.
It is the receptacle of all our karma, of all our actions
and impressions, which are ready to spring up into
visible forms. Every thought that we think, every deed
that we do, after a certain time becomes fine, goes into
seed form, so to speak, and lives in the fine body in a
potential form; and after a time it emerges again and
bears its results. These results condition the life of
man. Thus he moulds his own life. Man is not bound
by any other laws except those which he makes for
himself. Our thoughts, our words, and our deeds are
the threads of the net which we throw round ourselves, for good or for evil. Once we set in motion a

certain power, we have to take the full consequences of it. This is the law of karma.

Behind the subtle body lives the jiva, or individual soul of man. There are various discussions about the form and the size of this individual soul. According to some it is very small, like an atom; according to others it is not so small as that; according to still others it is very big, and so on. This jiva is a part of the universal substance, and it is also eternal; from time immemorial it has existed, and for time without end it will exist. It is passing through all these forms in order to manifest its real nature, which is purity. Every action that retards this manifestation is called an evil action; so also with thoughts. And every action and every thought that helps the jiva to expand, to manifest its real nature, is good. One theory that is held in common in India by the crudest dualists as well as by the most advanced non-dualists is that all the possibilities and powers of the soul are within it and do not come from any external source. They are in the soul in potential form, and our task is simply to manifest those potentialities.

The dualists also have the theory of reincarnation, which says that after the dissolution of this body, the jiva will have another, and after that has been dissolved, it will again have another, and so on, either here or in some other world. But this world is given the preference, since it is considered the best of all worlds for our purpose. Other worlds are conceived of as worlds where there is very little misery; but for that very reason, they argue, there is less chance of thinking of higher things there. Living in this world, which contains some happiness and a good deal of misery, the jiva some time or other gets awakened, as it were, and thinks of freeing itself. But just as very rich persons in this world have the least chance of thinking of higher things, so the jiva in heaven has little chance of progress; for its condition is the same as that of a rich man, only intensified. It has a very fine body, which knows no disease and is under no necessity of eating or drinking, and all its desires are fulfilled. The jiva lives there, having enjoyment after enjoyment, and so forgets all about its real nature.

But there are some souls in these higher worlds which, in spite of all the enjoyments, can evolve still further. Some dualists conceive of the goal as the highest heaven, where souls will live with God for ever. They will have beautiful bodies and will know neither disease nor death nor any other evil, and all their desires will be fulfilled. From time to time some of them will come back to this earth and take another body to teach human beings the way to God; and the great teachers of the world have been such. They were already free and were living with God in the highest sphere; but their love and sympathy for suffering humanity were so great that they incarnated themselves again to teach mankind the way to heaven.

Of course, we know that Advaita holds that this cannot be the goal or the ideal. Bodilessness must be the ideal. The ideal cannot be a finite existence. Anything short of the Infinite cannot be the ideal, and there cannot be an infinite body. That would be impossible, for the body comes from limitation. There cannot be infinite thought, because thought comes from limitation. We have to go beyond the body and beyond thought too, says Advaita. And we have also seen that, according to Advaita, this freedom is not to be attained; it is already ours. We only forget it and deny it. Perfection is not to be attained; it is already within us. Immortality and bliss are not to be acquired; we possess them already. They have been ours all the time. If you dare to declare that you are free, free you are this moment. If you say you are bound, bound you will remain. This is what Advaita boldly declares. I have told you the ideas of the dualists and other schools of philosophers. You can take whichever you like.

The highest ideal of Vedānta is very difficult to understand, and people are always quarrelling about it; and the greatest difficulty is that when they get hold of certain ideas they deny and fight other ideas. Take up what suits you and let others take up what they need. If you are desirous of clinging to this little individuality, to this limited manhood, remain in it, fulfil all these desires, and be content and pleased with them. If your experience of human life has been very good and nice, retain it as long as you like. And you can do so, for you are the makers of your own fortunes; none can compel you to give up your human life. You will be men as long as you like; none can prevent you. If you want to be angels, you will be angels. That is the law. But there may be others who do not even want to be angels. What right have you to think that theirs is a horrible notion? You may be frightened to lose a hundred pounds; but there may be others who would not even wink if they lost all the money they had in the world. There have been such men and there still are. Why do you dare to judge them according to your standards? You may cling to your limitations, and these little worldly ideas may be your highest ideal. You are welcome to them. It will be to you as you wish. But there are others who have seen the truth and cannot rest in these limitations, who have finished with these things and want to get beyond. The world with all its enjoyments is a mere mud-puddle for them. Why do you want to bind them down to your ideas? You must get rid of this tendency once for all. Accord a place to everyone.

I once read a story about some ships[1] that were caught in a cyclone in the South Sea Islands, and there was a picture of them in the *Illustrated London News.* All of them were wrecked except one English vessel, which weathered the storm. The picture showed the men who were going to be drowned, standing on the decks and cheering the people who were sailing through the storm. Be brave and generous like that. Do not drag others down to where you are.

Another foolish notion is that if we lose our little individuality there will be no morality, no hope for humanity. As if everybody had been dying for humanity all the time! God bless you! If in every country there were two hundred men and women really wanting to do good to humanity, the millennium would come in five days. We know how we are dying for humanity. This is all tall talk, and nothing else. The history of the world shows that those who never thought of their little individuality were the greatest

[1] H.M.S. *Calliope* and several American men-of-war at Samoa, in the Pacific Ocean.

benefactors of the human race, and that the more men and women think of themselves, the less they are able to do for others. One is unselfishness, and the other selfishness. Clinging to little enjoyments and desiring the continuation and repetition of this state of things are utter selfishness. They arise not from any desire for truth; their genesis is not in kindness for other beings, but in the utter selfishness of the human heart, in the idea, "I will have everything and do not care for anyone else." This is as it appears to me.

I should like to see more moral men in the world like some of those grand old prophets and sages of ancient times, who would have given up a hundred lives if by so doing they could benefit one little animal. Talk of morality and doing good to others! Silly talk of the present time! I should like to see moral men like Gautama Buddha, who did not believe in a Personal God or a personal soul, never asked about them, and was a perfect agnostic, and yet was ready to lay down his life for anyone, and worked all his life for the good of all, and thought only of the good of all. Well has it been said by his biographer, in describing his birth, that he was born for the good of the many, as a blessing to the many. He did not go to the forest to meditate for his own salvation; he felt that the world was burning and that he must find a way out. "Why is there so much misery in the world?"—was the one question that dominated his whole life. Do you think we are as moral as Buddha?

The more selfish a man, the more immoral he is. And so also with races. That race which has been the most self-centred has also been the most cruel and the

most wicked in the whole world. There has not been a
religion which has clung to dualism more intensely
than that founded by the Prophet of Arabia, and there
has not been a religion which has shed more blood and
been more cruel to others. In the Koran there is the
doctrine that a man who does not believe its teachings
should be killed—it is merciful to kill him! And the
surest way to get to heaven, where there are beautiful
houris and all sorts of sense enjoyments, is to kill these
unbelievers. Think of the bloodshed there has been in
consequence of such beliefs!

In the religion of Christ there was little of crudeness;
there is very little difference between the pure religion
of Christ and that of Vedānta. You find there the idea
of Oneness. But Christ also preached dualistic ideas
to the people in order to give them something tangible
to take hold of, to lead them up to the highest ideal.
The same Prophet who preached, "Our Father which
art in heaven," also preached, "I and my Father are
one," and the same Prophet knew that through the
"Father in heaven" lies the way to "I and my Father
are one." There was only blessing and love in the
religion of Christ. But as soon as crudeness crept in, it
was degraded into something not much better than the
religion of the Prophet of Arabia. It was crudeness
indeed, this fight for the little self, this clinging to
the "I," this desire not only for its preservation in this
life, but also for its continuance even after death. This
they declare to be unselfishness; this, the foundation
of morality! Lord help us, if this be the foundation of
morality! And strangely enough, men and women who
ought to know better think that all morality will be

destroyed if these little selves go, and stand aghast at the idea that morality can be based only on their destruction.

The watchword of all well-being, of all moral good, is "Not I but thou." Who cares whether there is a heaven or a hell, who cares if there is a soul or not, who cares if there is an Unchangeable or not? Here is the world, and it is full of misery. Go out into it as Buddha did and struggle to lessen its misery or die in the attempt. Forget yourselves—this is the first lesson to be learnt, whether you are a theist or an atheist, whether you are an agnostic or a Vedāntist, a Christian or a Mohammedan. The one lesson taught by all is the destruction of the little self and the building up of the Real Self.

Two forces have been working side by side in parallel lines. The one says "I," the other says "not I." Their manifestation is not only in man but in animals, not only in animals but in the smallest worms. The tigress that plunges her fangs into the warm blood of a human being would give up her own life to protect her cubs. The most depraved man, who thinks nothing of taking the lives of his brother men, will perhaps sacrifice himself without any hesitation to save his starving wife and children. Thus throughout creation these two forces are working side by side. Where you find the one, you find the other too. The one is selfishness; the other is unselfishness. The one is acquisition; the other is renunciation. The one takes; the other gives. From the lowest to the highest, the whole universe is the playground of these two forces. It does not require any demonstration; it is obvious to all.

What right has any section of the community to say that the working and the evolution of the universe are based upon one of these two factors alone—upon competition and struggle? What right has it to say that the whole working of the universe is based upon passion and fighting, upon competition and struggle? That these exist we do not deny; but what right has anyone to deny the working of the other force? Can any man deny that love—this "not I," this renunciation—is the only positive power in the universe? The other is only the misguided employment of the power of love. The wrong use of love brings competition; the real genesis of competition is in love. The real genesis of evil is in unselfishness. The creator of evil is good, and the end is also good. It is only misdirection of the power of good. A man who murders another is perhaps moved to do so by love of his own child. His love has become limited to that one little baby, to the exclusion of the millions of other human beings in the universe. Yet, limited or unlimited, it is the same love.

Thus the motive power of the whole universe, in whatever way it manifests itself, is that one wonderful thing, unselfishness, renunciation, love—the real, the only living force in existence. Therefore the Vedāntist insists upon oneness. We insist upon this explanation because we cannot admit two causes of the universe. If we simply hold that by limitation the same beautiful, wonderful love appears to be evil or vile, we find the whole universe explained by the one force of love. If not, two causes of the universe have to be taken for granted, one good and the other evil, one love and the other hatred. Which is more logical? Certainly the one-force theory.

Let us now pass on to things which do not possibly belong to dualism. I cannot stay longer with the dualists, I am afraid. My idea is to show that the highest ideal of morality and unselfishness goes hand in hand with the highest metaphysical conception, and that you need not lower your conception to get ethics and morality, but on the contrary, to reach a real basis of morality and ethics you must have the highest philosophical and scientific conceptions. Human knowledge is not antagonistic to human well-being. Indeed, it is knowledge alone that will save us in every department of life. Knowledge is worship. The more we know, the better for us.

Vedānta says that the cause of all that is apparently evil is the limitation of the Unlimited. The love which gets limited into little channels and seems to be evil eventually comes out at the other end and manifests itself as God. Vedānta also says that the cause of all this apparent evil is in ourselves. Do not blame any supernatural being; neither be hopeless and despondent, nor think we are in a place from which we can never escape unless someone comes and lends us a helping hand. That cannot be, says Vedānta. We are like silk-worms. We make the thread out of our own substance, and spin the cocoon, and in the course of time are imprisoned inside. But this cannot be for ever. We shall develop spiritual realization in that cocoon and, like the butterfly, come out free. We have woven this network of karma around ourselves, and in our ignorance we feel as if we are bound, and weep and

wail for help. But help does not come from without;
it comes from within ourselves.

Cry to all the gods in the universe. I cried for years,
and in the end I received help. But the help came from
within myself; and I had to undo what I had done by
mistake. That is the only way. I had to cut the net
which I had thrown round myself; and the power to do
this is within. Of this I am certain: that not one aspira-
tion in my life, well guided or ill guided, has been in
vain, but I am the resultant of all my past, both good
and evil. I have committed many mistakes in my life,
but mark you, I am sure that without every one of
those mistakes, I should not be what I am today; and
so I am quite satisfied to have made them. I do not
mean that you are to go home and wilfully commit
mistakes; do not misunderstand me in that way. But
do not mope because of the mistakes you have committed, but know that in the end all will come out
straight. It cannot be otherwise, because goodness is
our nature, purity is our nature, and that nature can
never be destroyed. Our essential nature always remains the same.

What we must understand is that what we call mistakes, or evil, we commit because we are weak, and
we are weak because we are ignorant. I prefer to call
them mistakes. The word *sin*, although originally a
very good word, has a certain flavour about it that
frightens me. Who makes us ignorant? We ourselves.
We put our hands over our eyes and weep because it
is dark. Take the hands away and there is light; the
light exists always for us, the self-effulgent nature of
the human soul. Do you not hear what your modern

scientific men say? What is the cause of evolution? Desire. The animal wants to do something, but does not find the environment favourable and therefore develops a new body. Who develops it? The animal itself—its will. You have developed from the lowest amoeba. Continue to exercise your will and it will take you higher still. The will is almighty. If it is almighty, you may say, why can I not do everything I like? But you are thinking only of your little self. Look back on yourselves from the state of the amoeba to the human being. Who made all that? Your own will. Can you deny, then, that will is almighty? That which has made you come up so high can make you go higher still. What you want is character, strengthening of the will.

If I teach you, therefore, that your nature is evil, that you should go home and sit in sackcloth and ashes and weep your lives out because you took certain false steps, it will not help you, but will weaken you all the more, and I shall be showing you the road to more evil than good. If this room has been full of darkness for thousands of years and you come in and begin to weep and wail, "Oh, the darkness!"—will the darkness vanish? Strike a match and light comes in a moment. What good will it do you to think all your lives, "Oh, I have done evil; I have made many mistakes"? It requires no ghost to tell us that. Bring in the light and the evil goes in a moment. Build up your character and manifest your real nature, the Effulgent, the Resplendent, the Ever Pure, and call it up in everyone that you see.

I wish that every one of us had come to such a state

that even in the vilest of human beings we could see
the Real Self within, and instead of condemning them,
say: "Rise, Thou Effulgent One! Rise, Thou who art
always pure! Rise, Thou Birthless and Deathless One!
Rise, Almighty One! and manifest Thy true nature.
These little manifestations do not befit Thee." This is
the highest prayer that Advaita teaches. This is the
only prayer—to remember our true nature, the God
who is always within us, thinking of it always as
infinite, almighty, ever good, ever beneficent, selfless,
bereft of all limitations; and to remember that because
that nature is selfless, it is strong and fearless; for only
to the selfish comes fear. He who has nothing to desire
for himself—whom does he fear and what can frighten
him? What fear has death for him? What fear has evil
for him? So if we are Advaitists, we must think from
this moment that our old self is dead and gone. The
old Mr., Mrs., and Miss So-and-so are gone. They
were mere superstitions; and what remains is the Ever
Pure, the Ever Strong, the Almighty, the All-knowing
—That alone remains for us. And then all fear vanishes from us. Who can injure us, the Omnipresent?
All weakness has vanished from us; and our only work
is to arouse this knowledge in our fellow beings. We
see that they too are the same Pure Self, only they do
not know it. We must teach them; we must help them
to rouse up their infinite nature. This is what I feel
to be absolutely necessary all over the world.

These doctrines are old—older, possibly, than many
mountains. All truth is eternal. Truth is nobody's
property; no race, no individual, can lay exclusive
claim to it. Truth is the nature of all souls. Who can

lay special claim to it? But it has to be made practical, to be made simple (for the highest truths are always simple), so that it may penetrate every pore of human society and become the property of the highest intellects and the commonest minds, of man, woman, and child at the same time. All these ratiocinations of logic, all these bundles of metaphysics, all these theologies and ceremonies, may have been good in their own time. But let us try to make things simpler and bring about the golden days when every man will be a worshipper, and the Reality in every man will be the object of worship.

THE WAY TO THE REALIZATION OF
THE UNIVERSAL RELIGION

(Delivered in the Universalist Church, Pasadena, California, January 28, 1900)

NO SEARCH HAS BEEN DEARER to the human heart than that which brings to us light from God. No study has taken so much human energy, whether in times past or present, as the study of the soul, of God, and of human destiny. However deeply immersed we are in our daily occupations, in our ambitions, in our work, sometimes in the midst of the greatest of our struggles there comes a pause; the mind stops and wants to know something beyond this world. Sometimes it catches glimpses of a realm beyond the senses, and a struggle to get at it is the result. Thus it has been throughout the ages in all countries. Man has wanted to look beyond, wanted to expand himself; and all that we call progress, evolution, has always been measured by that one search, the search for human destiny, the search for God.

As our social struggles are represented, among different nations, by different social organizations, so man's spiritual struggles are represented by various religions. And as different social organizations are constantly quarrelling, are constantly at war with each other, so these spiritual organizations have been constantly at war with each other, constantly quarrelling. Men belonging to a particular social organization claim that the right to live belongs only to them, and so long as they can, they want to exercise that right at the cost of the weak. We know that just now there is a fierce struggle of that sort going on in South Africa.[1] Similarly each religious sect has claimed the exclusive right to live. And thus we find that though nothing has brought man more blessings than religion, yet at the same time there is nothing that has brought him more horror than religion. Nothing has made more for peace and love than religion; nothing has engendered fiercer hatred than religion. Nothing has made the brotherhood of man more tangible than religion; nothing has bred more bitter enmity between man and man than religion. Nothing has built more charitable institutions, more hospitals for men and even for animals, than religion; nothing has deluged the world with more blood than religion.

We know, at the same time, that there has always been an opposing undercurrent of thought; there have always been parties of men, philosophers, students of comparative religion, who have tried and are still trying to bring about harmony in the midst of all these jarring and discordant sects. As regards certain countries these attempts have succeeded, but as regards the whole world they have failed. Then again, there are some religions, which have come down to us from the remotest antiquity, imbued with the idea that all sects should be allowed to live—that every sect has a meaning, a great idea, imbedded in it, and therefore all sects are necessary for the good of the world and ought to be helped. In modern times the same idea is prevalent,

[1] A reference to the Boer War.

and attempts are made from time to time to reduce it
to practice. But these attempts do not always come up
to our expectations, up to the required efficiency. Nay,
to our great disappointment, we sometimes find that
we are quarrelling all the more.

Now, leaving aside dogmatic study and taking a
common-sense view of the thing, we find at the start
that there is a tremendous life-power in all the great
religions of the world. Some may say that they are
unaware of this; but ignorance is no excuse. If a man
says, "I do not know what is going on in the external
world, therefore the things that are said to be going on
there do not exist," that plea is inexcusable. Now,
those of you who are watching the movement of religious thought all over the world are perfectly aware
that not one of the great religions of the world has died.
Not only so; each one of them is progressing. The
Christians are multiplying, the Mohammedans are
multiplying, and the Hindus are gaining ground; the
Jews also are increasing in numbers, and as a result of
their activities all over the world, the fold of Judaism
is constantly expanding.

Only one religion of the world—an ancient, great
religion—is dwindling away, and that is the religion of
Zoroastrianism, the religion of the ancient Persians.
After the Mohammedan conquest of Persia, about a
hundred thousand of these people came to India and
took shelter there, and some remained in Persia. Those
who were in Persia, under the constant persecution of
the Mohammedans, dwindled till there are at most only
ten thousand. In India there are about eighty thousand
of them, but they do not increase. Of course, there is

an initial difficulty: they do not convert others to their religion. And then, this handful of persons living in India, with the pernicious custom of cousin-marriage, does not multiply. With this single exception, all the great religions are living, spreading, and increasing.

We must remember that all the great religions of the world are very ancient—not one has been formed at the present time—and that every religion of the world had its origin in the region between the Ganges and the Euphrates. Not one great religion has arisen in Europe; not one in America—not one. Every religion is of Asiatic origin and belongs to that part of the world. If what the modern scientists say is true, that the survival of the fittest is the test, these religions prove by their still being alive that they are yet fit for some people. And there is a reason why they should live: they bring good to many. Look at the Mohammedans, how they are spreading in some places in southern Asia, and spreading like wildfire in Africa. The Buddhists are spreading over central Asia all the time. The Hindus, like the Jews, do not convert others; still, gradually other races are coming within Hinduism and adopting the manners and customs of the Hindus and falling into line with them. Christianity, you all know, is spreading—though I am not sure that the results are equal to the energy put forth. The Christians' attempt at propaganda has one tremendous defect, and that is the defect of all Western institutions: the machine consumes ninety per cent of the energy; there is too much machinery. Preaching has always been the business of the Asiatics. The Western people are grand in organization—social institutions,

armies, governments, and so forth. But when it comes
to preaching religion, they cannot come near the Asiatics, whose business it has been all the time—and
they know it, and do not use too much machinery.

This, then, is a fact in the present history of the
human race: that all these great religions exist and
are spreading and multiplying. Now, there is a meaning, certainly, to this; and had it been the will of an
all-wise and all-merciful Creator that one of these
religions should alone exist and the rest die, it would
have become a fact long, long ago. If it were a fact that
only one of these religions was true and all the rest
were false, by this time it would have covered the
whole world. But this is not so; not one has gained all
the ground. All religions sometimes advance, sometimes decline. Now, just think of this: in your own
country there are more than sixty millions of people,
and only twenty-one millions profess a religion of
some sort. So it is not always progress. In every country, probably, if the statistics were taken, you would
find that the religions sometimes progress and sometimes go back. Sects are multiplying all the time. If
the claim of any one religion that it has all the truth,
and that God has given it all that truth in a certain
book, be true, why then are there so many sects? Not
fifty years pass before there are twenty sects founded
upon the same book. If God has put all the truth in
certain books, He does not give us those books in order
that we may quarrel over texts. That seems to be the
fact. Why is this? Even if a book were given by God
which contained all the truth about religion, it would
not serve the purpose, because nobody could under-

stand the book. Take the Bible, for instance, and all
the sects that exist among the Christians. Each one
puts its own interpretation upon the same text, and
each says that it alone understands that text and all
the rest are wrong. So with every religion. There are
many sects among the Mohammedans and among the
Buddhists, and hundreds among the Hindus.

Now, I place these facts before you in order to show
you that any attempt to bring all humanity to one
method of thinking in spiritual things has been a
failure and always will be a failure. Every man who
starts a theory, even at the present day, finds that if
he goes twenty miles away from his followers they will
make twenty sects. You see that happening all the time.
You cannot make all conform to the same ideas; that
is a fact, and I thank God that it is so. I am not against
any sect. I am glad that sects exist, and I only wish
they may go on multiplying more and more. Why?
Simply because of this: If you and I and all who are
present here were to think exactly the same thoughts,
there would be no thoughts for us to think. We know
that two or more forces must come into collision in
order to produce motion. It is the clash of thought,
the differentiation of thought, that awakens thought.
Now, if we all thought alike, we should be like Egyp-
tian mummies in a museum, looking vacantly at one
another's faces—no more than that. Whirls and eddies
occur only in a rushing, living stream. There are no
whirlpools in stagnant, dead water.

When religions are dead, there will be no more
sects; it will be the perfect peace and harmony of the
grave. But so long as mankind thinks, there will be

sects. Variation is the sign of life, and it must be there. I pray that sects may multiply so that at last there will be as many sects as human beings and each one will have his own method, his individual method of thought, in religion.

Such a situation, however, exists already. Each one of us is thinking in his own way. But this natural thinking has been obstructed all the time and is still being obstructed. If the sword is not used directly, other means are used. Just hear what one of the best preachers in New York says. He preaches that the Filipinos should be conquered because that is the only way to teach Christianity to them! They are already Catholics; but he wants to make them Presbyterians, and for this he is ready to lay all this terrible sin of bloodshed upon his race. How terrible! And this man is one of the greatest preachers of this country, one of the best informed men. Think of the state of the world when a man like that is not ashamed to stand up and utter such arrant nonsense; and think of the state of the world when an audience cheers him. Is this civilization? It is the old blood-thirstiness of the tiger, the cannibal, the savage, coming out once more under new names in new circumstances. What else can it be? If such is the state of things now, think of the horrors through which the world passed in olden times, when every sect was trying, by every means in its power, to tear to pieces the other sects. History shows that the tiger in us is only asleep; it is not dead. When opportunities come it jumps up and, as of old, uses its claws and fangs. And apart from the sword, apart from material weapons, there are weapons still more terrible: contempt, social hatred, and social ostracism.

Now, these afflictions that are hurled against persons who do not think exactly in the same way we do are the most terrible of all afflictions. And why should everybody think just as we do? I do not see any reason. If I am a rational man, I should be glad that they do not think just as I do. I do not want to live in a grave-like land. I want to be a man in a world of men. Thinking beings must differ; difference is the first sign of thought. If I am a thoughtful man, certainly I ought to like to live among thoughtful persons, where there are differences of opinion.

Then arises the question: How can all this variety be true? If one thing is true, its negation is false. How can contradictory opinions be true at the same time? This is the question which I intend to answer. But I shall first ask you: Are all the religions of the world really contradictory? I do not mean the external forms in which great thoughts are clad. I do not mean the different buildings, languages, rituals, books, and so forth, employed in various religions, but I mean the internal soul of every religion. Every religion has a soul behind it, and that soul may differ from the soul of another religion; but are they contradictory? Do they contradict or supplement each other?—that is the question.

I took up this question when I was quite a boy, and have been studying it all my life. Thinking that my conclusion may be of some help to you, I place it before you. I believe that they are not contradictory; they are supplementary. Each religion, as it were, takes up one

part of the great, universal truth and spends its whole
force in embodying and typifying that part of the
great truth. It is therefore addition, not exclusion. That
is the idea. System after system arises, each one embodying a great ideal; ideals must be added to ideals.
And this is how humanity marches on.

Man never progresses from error to truth, but from
truth to truth—from lesser truth to higher truth, but
never from error to truth. The child may develop more
than the father; but was the father inane? The child
is the father plus something else. If your present stage
of knowledge is much higher than the stage you were
in when you were a child, would you look down upon
that earlier stage now? Will you look back and call it
inanity? Your present stage is the knowledge of childhood plus something more.

Then again, we know that there may be almost
contradictory points of view of a thing, but they all
point to the same thing. Suppose a man is journeying
towards the sun and as he advances he takes a photo-
graph of the sun at every stage. When he comes back,
he has many photographs of the sun, which he places
before us. We see that no two are alike; and yet who
will deny that all these are photographs of the same
sun, from different standpoints? Take four photographs
of this church from different corners. How different
they would look! And yet they would all represent this
church. In the same way, we are all looking at truth
from different standpoints, which vary according to our
birth, education, surroundings, and so on. We are
viewing truth, getting as much of it as these circumstances will permit, colouring it with our own feelings,

understanding it with our own intellects, and grasping it with our own minds. We can know only as much of truth as is related to us, as much of it as we are able to receive. This makes the difference between man and man and sometimes even occasions contradictory ideas. Yet we all belong to the same great, universal truth.

My idea, therefore, is that all these religions are different forces in the economy of God, working for the good of mankind, and that not one can become dead, not one can be killed. Just as you cannot kill any force in nature, so you cannot kill any one of these spiritual forces. You have seen that each religion is living. From time to time it may retrogress or go forward. At one time it may be shorn of a good many of its trappings; at another time it may be covered with all sorts of trappings. But all the same, the soul is ever there; it can never be lost. The ideal which every religion represents is never lost, and so every religion is intelligently on the march.

And that universal religion about which philosophers and others have dreamt in every country already exists. It is here. As the universal brotherhood of man already exists, so also does the universal religion. Which of you that have travelled far and wide have not found brothers and sisters in every nation? I have found them all over the world. Brotherhood already exists; only there are numbers of persons who fail to see this and upset it by crying for new brotherhoods. The universal religion, too, already exists. If the priests and other people who have taken upon themselves the task of preaching different religions simply cease preaching for a few moments, we shall see it is there.

They are disturbing it all the time, because it is to their interest.

You see that the priests in every country are very conservative. Why is this so? There are very few priests who lead the people; most of them are led by the people and are their slaves and servants. If you say it is dry, they say it is dry; if you say it is black, they say it is black. If the people advance, the priests must advance. They cannot lag behind. So before blaming the priests—it is the fashion to blame the priests—you ought to blame yourselves. You get only what you deserve. What would be the fate of a priest who wanted to give you new and advanced ideas and lead you forward? His children would probably starve and he would be clad in rags. He is governed by the same worldly laws that you are governed by. If you move on, he says, "Let us march."

Of course, there are exceptional souls, not cowed by public opinion. They see the truth, and truth alone they value. Truth has got hold of them, has got possession of them, as it were, and they cannot but march ahead. They never look backward. And they do not pay heed to people. God alone exists for them; He is the light before them and they are following that light.

I met a Mormon gentleman in this country who tried to convert me to his faith. I said: "I have great respect for your opinions, but in certain points we do not agree. I belong to a monastic order, and you believe in marrying many wives. But why don't you go to India to preach?" He was simply astonished. He said, "Why, you don't believe in any marriage at all, and we believe in polygamy, and yet you ask me to go to your country!" I said: "Yes. My countrymen will hear any religious thought, wherever it may come from. I wish you would go to India. First, because I am a great believer in sects. Secondly, there arc many men in India who are not at all satisfied with any of the existing sects, and on account of this dissatisfaction they will not have anything to do with religion; and possibly you might get some of them."

The greater the number of sects, the more chance of people's becoming religious. In a hotel, where there are all sorts of food, everyone has a chance to have his appetite satisfied. So I want sects to multiply in every country, that more people may have a chance to be spiritual.

Do not think that people do not like religion. I do not believe that. The preachers cannot give them what they need. The same man who may have been branded as an atheist, as a materialist, or what not, may meet a man who gives him the truth needed by him, and he may turn out to be the most spiritual man in the community. We can eat only in our own way. For instance, we Hindus eat with our fingers. Our fingers are suppler than yours; you cannot use your fingers the same way. Not only should the food be supplied; it should also be taken in your own particular way. Not only must you have the spiritual ideas; they must also come to you according to your own method. They must speak your own language, the language of your soul, and then alone will they satisfy you. When the man comes who speaks my language and gives me the truth in my language, I at once understand it and receive it for ever. This is a great fact.

Now, from this we see that there are various grades
and types of human minds—and what a task the religions take upon themselves! A man brings forth two
or three doctrines and claims that his religion ought
to satisfy all humanity. He goes out into the world,
God's menagerie, with a little cage in hand, and says:
"Man and the elephant and everybody have to fit into
this. Even if we have to cut the elephant into pieces,
he must go in." Again, there may be a sect with a few
good ideas. It says, "All men must come in!" "But there
is no room for them." "Never mind! Cut them to pieces;
get them in anyhow; if they don't get in, why, they
will be damned." No preacher, no sect, have I ever
met that paused and asked, "Why is it that people do
not listen to us?" Instead they curse them and say,
"The people are wicked." They never ask: "How is
it that people do not listen to my words? Why can I
not make them see the truth? Why can I not speak in
their language? Why can I not open their eyes?"
Surely they ought to know better, and when they find
that people do not listen to them, if they curse anybody it should be themselves. But it is always the
people's fault! They never try to make their sect large
enough to embrace everyone.

Therefore we at once see why there has been so
much narrow-mindedness, the part always claiming to
be the whole, the little, finite unit always laying claim
to the infinite. Think of little sects, born only a few
hundred years ago, out of fallible human brains, making this arrogant claim of knowing the whole of God's
infinite truth! Think of the arrogance of it! If it shows
anything, it shows how vain human beings are. And

it is no wonder that such claims have always failed, and by the mercy of the Lord are always destined to fail. In this line the Mohammedans were the best off. Every step forward was made with the sword—the Koran in the one hand and the sword in the other: "Take the Koran, or you must die. There is no other alternative!" You know from history how phenomenal was their success; for six hundred years nothing could resist them. And then there came a time when they had to cry halt. So will it be with other religions if they follow the same methods.

We are such babies! We always forget human nature. When we begin life we think that our fate will be something extraordinary, and nothing can make us disbelieve that. But when we grow old we think differently. So with religions. In their early stages, when they spread a little, they get the idea that they can change the minds of the whole human race in a few years, and they go on killing and massacring to make converts by force. Then they fail and begin to understand better. These religions did not succeed in what they started out to do, which was a great blessing. Just think! If one of those fanatical sects had succeeded all over the world, where would man be today? The Lord be blessed that they did not succeed! Yet each one represents a great truth; each religion represents a particular excellence, something which is its soul.

There is an old story which comes to my mind: There were some ogresses who used to kill people and do all sorts of mischief; but they themselves could not be killed until someone should find out that their souls were in certain birds and so long as the birds were

alive nothing could destroy the ogresses. So each one
of us has, as it were, such a bird, where his soul is—
has an ideal, a mission to perform in life. Every human
being is an embodiment of such an ideal, such a mission. Whatever else you may lose, so long as that ideal
is not lost and that mission is not hurt, nothing can
kill you. Wealth may come and go, misfortunes may
be piled mountain high, but if you have kept the ideal
pure, nothing can kill you. You may have grown old,
even a hundred years old, but if that mission is fresh
and young in your heart, what can kill you? But when
that ideal is lost and that mission is forgotten, nothing
can save you. All the wealth, all the power of the
world will not save you.

And what are nations but multiplied individuals?
So each nation has a mission of its own to perform in
this harmony of races, and so long as a nation keeps
to that ideal, nothing can kill that nation. But if the
nation gives up its mission and goes after something
else, its life becomes short and ultimately it vanishes.

And so with religions. The fact that all these old
religions are living today proves that they must have
kept that mission intact. In spite of all their mistakes,
in spite of all difficulties, in spite of all quarrels, in
spite of all the incrustation of forms and rituals, the
heart of every one of them is sound—it is a throbbing,
beating, living heart. They have not lost, any of them,
the great mission they came for. And it is splendid to
study that mission. Take Mohammedanism, for instance. Christian people hate no religion in the world
so much as Mohammedanism. They think it is the very
worst form of religion that ever existed. But as soon as

a man becomes a Mohammedan, the whole of Islām receives him as a brother with open arms, without making any distinction, which no other religion does. If one of your American Indians became a Mohammedan, the Sultan of Turkey would have no objection to dining with him. If he had brains, no position would be barred to him. In this country I have never yet seen a church where the white man and the Negro can kneel side by side to pray. Just think of that: Islām makes its followers all equal. So that, you see, is the peculiar excellence of Mohammedanism. In many places in the Koran you find very sensual ideals of life. Never mind. What Mohammedanism comes to preach to the world is this practical brotherhood of all belonging to their faith. That is the essential part of the Mohammedan religion; and all the other ideas, about heaven and life and so forth, are not real Mohammedanism. They are accretions.

With the Hindus you will find one great idea: spirituality. In no other religion, in no other sacred books in the world, will you find so much energy spent in defining the idea of God. They tried to describe God in such a way that no earthly touch might mar Him. The Spirit must be divine; and Spirit, as such, must not be identified with the physical world. The idea of unity, of the realization of God, the Omnipresent, is preached throughout. They think it is nonsense to say that God lives in heaven, and all that. That is a mere human, anthropomorphic idea. All the heaven that ever existed is now and here. One moment in infinite time is quite as good as any other moment. If you believe in a God, you can see Him even now. We

Hindus think that religion begins when you have realized something. It is not believing in doctrines or giving intellectual assent or making declarations. If there is a God, have you seen Him? If you say no, then what right have you to believe in Him? If you are in doubt whether there is a God, why do you not struggle to see Him? Why do you not renounce the world and spend the whole of your life for this one object? Renunciation and spirituality are the two great ideals of India, and it is because India clings to these ideals that all her mistakes count for so little.

With the Christians, the central idea that has been preached by them is the same: "Watch and pray, for the kingdom of heaven is at hand"—which means: Purify your minds and be ready. You recollect that the Christians, even in the darkest days, even in the most superstitious Christian countries, have always tried to prepare themselves for the coming of the Lord by trying to help others, building hospitals, and so on. So long as the Christians keep to that ideal, their religion lives.

Now, an ideal presents itself to my mind. It may be only a dream. I do not know whether it will ever be realized in this world; but sometimes it is better to dream a dream than to die on hard facts. Great truths, even in a dream, are good—better than bad facts. So let us dream a dream.

You know that there are various grades of mind. You may be a matter-of-fact, common-sense rationalist. You do not care for forms and ceremonies; you want intellectual, hard, ringing facts, and they alone will satisfy you. Then there are the Puritans and the Mohammedans, who will not allow a picture or a statue in their place of worship. Very well. But there is another man who is more artistic. He wants a great deal of art—beauty of lines and curves, colours, flowers, forms; he wants candles, lights, and all the insignia and paraphernalia of ritual, that he may see God. His mind grasps God in those forms, as yours grasps Him through the intellect. Then there is the devotional man, whose soul is crying for God; he has no other idea but to worship God and praise Him. Then again, there is the philosopher, standing outside all these things, mocking at them. He thinks: "What nonsense they are! What ideas about God!"

They may laugh at each other, but each one has a place in this world. All these various minds, all these various types, are necessary. If there is ever going to be an ideal religion, it must be broad and large enough to supply food for all these minds. It must supply the strength of philosophy to the philosopher, the de-votee's heart to the worshipper; to the ritualist it must give all that the most marvellous symbolism can con-vey; to the poet it must give as much of heart as he can absorb, and other things besides. To make such a broad religion, we shall have to go back to the very source and take them all in.

Our watchword, then, will be acceptance and not exclusion. Not only toleration; for so-called toleration is often blasphemy and I do not believe in it. I believe in acceptance. Why should I tolerate? Toleration means that I think that you are wrong and I am just allowing you to live. Is it not blasphemy to think that you and I are allowing others to live? I accept all the religions that were in the past and worship with them all; I worship God with every one of them, in whatever form they worship Him. I shall go to the mosque of the Mohammedan; I shall enter the Christian church and kneel before the Crucifix; I shall enter the Buddhist temple, where I shall take refuge in Buddha and his Law. I shall go into the forest and sit down in meditation with the Hindu, who is trying to see the Light which enlightens the hearts of everyone.

Not only shall I do all this, but I shall keep my heart open for all the religions that may come in the future. Is God's Book finished? Or is revelation still going on? It is a marvellous Book—these spiritual revelations of the world. The Bible, the Vedas, the Koran, and all other sacred books are but so many pages, and an infinite number of pages remain yet to be unfolded. I shall leave my heart open for all of them. We stand in the present, but open ourselves to the infinite future. We take in all that has been in the past, enjoy the light of the present, and open every window of the heart for all that will come in the future. Salutation to all the prophets of the past, to all the great ones of the present, and to all that are to come in the future!

GLOSSARY

GLOSSARY

Advaita   Non-duality; a school of Vedānta philosophy teaching the oneness of God, soul, and universe, whose chief exponent was Śankarāchārya (A.D. 788-820).

ākāśa   The first of the five material elements that constitute the universe; often translated as "space" and "ether." The four other elements are vāyu (air), agni (fire), ap (water), and prithivi (earth).

Arjuna   A hero of the epic *Mahābhārata* and a friend and disciple of Krishna.

aśvattha tree   The holy fig tree; sometimes used as a symbol of the universe.

Ātman   The Self or Soul; denotes both the Supreme Soul and the individual soul, which. according to Non-dualistic Vedānta, are ultimately identical.

Bhagavad Gitā   An important Hindu scripture, comprising eighteen chapters of the epic *Mahābhārata* and containing the teachings of Śri Krishna.

Bo-tree   The famous tree under which Buddha attained illumination.

Brahmā   The Creator God; the First Person of the Hindu Trinity, the other two being Vishnu and Śiva.

Brahmaloka   The plane of Brahmā, roughly corresponding to the highest heaven of the dualistic religions, where fortunate souls go after death and enjoy communion with the Personal God.

Brahman   The Absolute; the Supreme Reality of the Vedānta philosophy.

309

310

Brāhmana   That portion of the Vedas which gives the rules for the employment of the hymns at the various sacrifices, their origin and detailed explanation, etc. It is distinct from the Mantra portion of the Vedas, which contains the collection of hymns used in the sacrifices.

brāhmin   A member of the priestly caste, the highest caste in Hindu society.

buddhi   The determinative faculty of the mind, which makes decisions; sometimes translated as "intellect."

Chārvākas   Followers of Chārvāka, an atheistic philosopher who denied the existence of God, soul, and hereafter and repudiated the authority of the Vedas.

Chhāndogya Upanishad   One of the major Upanishads. See Upanishads.

chitta   The mind-stuff; that part of the inner organ which is the storehouse of memory or which seeks for pleasurable objects.

cycle   A world period, representing the duration of the universe between its manifestation and its return to the unmanifested state.

devas   (Lit., shining ones.) The gods of Hindu mythology.

Gitā   Same as Bhagavad Gitā.

guru   Spiritual preceptor.

Indra   The king of the gods.

indriyas   The sense-organs, consisting of the five organs of perception, the five organs of action, and the mind.

Iśa Upanishad   One of the major Upanishads. See Upanishads.

jiva   (Lit., living being.) The individual soul, which in essence is one with the Universal Soul.

jivanmukta   One who has attained liberation while living in the body.

Kapila   The founder of the Sāmkhya philosophy.

karma   Action in general; duty. The Vedas use the word chiefly to denote ritualistic worship and humanitarian action.

Katha Upanishad   One of the major Upanishads. See Upanishads.

Krishna   An Incarnation of God described in the *Mahābhārata* and the *Bhāgavata*.

mahat   The cosmic mind.

Manu   The celebrated ancient lawgiver of India.

māyā   A term of the Vedānta philosophy denoting ignorance obscuring the vision of Reality; the cosmic illusion on account of which the One appears as many, the Absolute as the relative.

māyāvādin   A believer in the doctrine of māyā.

Nirvāna   Final absorption in Brahman, or the All-pervading Reality, through the annihilation of the individual ego.

prāna   The vital breath, which sustains life in a physical body; the primal energy or force, of which other physical forces are manifestations. Prāna is also a name of Saguna Brahman, or Brahman with attributes.

Purānas   Books of Hindu mythology.

rāja-yoga   A system of yoga ascribed to Patanjali, dealing with concentration and its methods, control of the mind, samādhi, and similar matters.

Rig-Veda   One of the four Vedas. See Vedas.

Samhitā   A section of the Vedas containing a collection of hymns.

Sāmkhya   One of the six systems of orthodox Hindu philosophy, which teaches that the universe evolves as the result of the union of prakriti (nature) and Purusha (Spirit). It was founded by Kapila.

samskāra   Mental impression or tendency created by an action.

Śankarāchārya   One of the greatest saints and philosophers of India, the foremost exponent of Advaita Vedānta (A.D. 788-820).

sannyāsin   A Hindu monk who has renounced the world in order to realize God.

Śri   The word is often used as an honorific prefix to the names of deities and eminent persons, or of celebrated books generally of a sacred character; sometimes used as an auspicious sign at the commencement of letters, manuscripts, etc., also as an equivalent of the English term *Mr.*

Śvetāśvatara Upanishad   One of the major Upanishads. See Upanishads.

Swami   (Lit., lord.) A title of the monks belonging to the Vedānta school.

Tat tvam asi   (Lit., "That thou art.") A sacred formula of the Vedas denoting the identity of the individual self and the Supreme Self.

Upanishads   The well-known Hindu scriptures containing the philosophy of the Vedas. They are one hundred and eight in number, of which eleven are called major Upanishads.

Varuna   A Vedic deity; the presiding deity of the ocean.

Vedānta   (Lit., the essence or concluding part of the

Vedas.) A system of philosophy mainly based upon the teachings of the Upanishads, the Bhagavad Gitā, and the *Brahma Sutras.*

Vedas   The revealed scriptures of the Hindus, consisting of the Rig-Veda, Sāma-Veda, Yajur-Veda, and Atharva-Veda.

yoga   Union of the individual soul and the Supreme Soul. The discipline by which such union is effected. The Yoga system of philosophy, ascribed to Patanjali, is one of the six systems of orthodox Hindu philosophy, and deals with the realization of Truth through the control of the mind.

yogi   One who practises yoga.

Yudhishthira   The eldest of the five sons of Pāndu; one of the heroes of the Mahābhārata.

INDEX

INDEX

Absolute, 59. *See also* Brahman
ākāśa, 178-79, 252
Ātman, *see* Soul

Bhagavad Gitā, 105
body, 12
Brahmaloka, 99, 185
Brahman, 75, 167, 172, 232. *See also* God (Impersonal) and Soul
Buddha, 29, 56, 68, 281

cause: same as effect, 125, 127, 155
Chārvākas, 56-7
Christ, 282
Christianity, 293-94: message of, 306
cycle, 127, 178

death, 14, 29-30, 198-99
deluge, 4
desire: cause of misery, 79, 81
dualism, 109, 183, 275 ff.

ethics: of Vedānta, 224-25; 255; monistic basis of, 260

evil, 75-76. *See also* good and evil
evolution, 6-7, 33, 91, 128 ff., 153 ff., 274, 287

faith, 219-20
fanaticism, 40
Ferris wheel, 157, 175
freedom, 42, 57, 69 ff.

God: evolution of, 47, 51, 54; embodiment of freedom, 69; 73, 75; in everything, 77-8, 80, 82, 85; 81, 128; is intelligence, 130, 158; 131, 132, 150, 175; Impersonal, 242, 243, 245, 258-59, 263-65; Personal, 254-55, 258-59, 263-65
gods, 89-90
good and evil, 33 ff., 35-6, 90 ff.

heaven, 238
hell, 240, 241
heredity, 146-48
Hinduism: message of, 305

immortality, 90, 152 ff.

315